This Book Will Change Your Mind About Mental Health

Nathan Filer is a *The Shock of the Fall*, his novel about the life of a young man grieving the loss of his brother, was a *Sunday Times* bestseller and has been translated into thirty languages. It won the Costa Book of the Year, the Betty Trask Prize, the National Book Award for Popular Fiction and the Writers' Guild Award for Best First Novel. He has written for the *Guardian* and the *New York Times*. His BBC Radio 4 documentary, *The Mind in the Media*, which explored portrayals of mental illness in fiction and journalism, was shortlisted for a Mind Media Award. He lives in Bristol with his wife and two children.

Further praise for *This Book Will Change Your Mind About Mental Health*:

'Schizophrenia has been called the heartland of modern psychiatry because the quest to understand and treat it has come almost to define the discipline . . . Absorbing . . . Filer does a brilliant job of bringing order and humanity to a seemingly chaotic scene.' Paul Broks, *Literary Review*

'A hard-hitting and thoughtful account of contemporary mental health practices . . . Mental health is "messy and chaotic" but that doesn't mean we shouldn't keep trying to make sense of it. This impressive book advocates that we all need to be part of the conversation.' Ian Critchley, *Sunday Times*

'I find F t terrain appealin: h from a

book so short on definitive answers. Filer's humility for himself and his professions seems fitting . . . The tone remains questing and buoyant even as we move through lives devastated by so-called schizophrenia. I hope it will be widely read and discussed.' Cathy Rentzenbrink, *The Times*

'Through a distinctive style of writing that is at once conversational, confiding and challenging, he helps us open our minds to new ways of thinking about mental health, about each other, and about our own selves . . . It reminds us that, in many respects, when it comes to what goes on in our heads, we are all on the same human continuum.' *Bookseller* Book of the Month

'This moving, endlessly quotable, and extremely thought-provoking book will hopefully do just that . . . It feels like a gift to us all, a gift whose importance cannot be exaggerated, and whose potential we all could help to realise.' Bristol 24/7

'These true stories are fascinating, harrowing and widely varied in their outcomes . . . His argument is humane, cogent and, well, sane.' Charlotte Moore, *Oldie*

'In his first-person stories, Filer brings his novelist's eye for detail into play . . . The stories are all the more compelling as they are enriched by Filer's own personal experience as a nurse.' Rachel Kelly, *The Tablet*

---

by the same author

The Shock of the Fall

This
Book
will
Change
Your
Mind
about
Mental
Health

A journey into
the heartland of psychiatry

Nathan
Filer

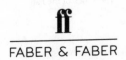
FABER & FABER

First published in 2019
by Faber & Faber Limited
Bloomsbury House
74–77 Great Russell Street
London WC1B 3DA
This paperback edition published in 2020

Typeset by Typo•glyphix
Printed and bound by CPI Group (UK) Ltd, Croydon, CR0 4YY

The right of Nathan Filer to be identified as author of this work
has been asserted in accordance with Section 77 of the Copyright,
Designs and Patents Act 1988

This Book Will Change Your Mind About Mental Health was previously published in
hardback under the title *The Heartland*.

*This book is sold subject to the condition that it shall not, by way of trade or otherwise, be
lent, resold, hired out or otherwise circulated without the publisher's prior consent in any
form of binding or cover other than that in which it is published and without a similar
condition including this condition being imposed on the subsequent purchaser*

A CIP record for this book
is available from the British Library

ISBN 978-0-571-34597-7

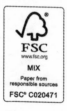

To S.R.C

Contents

A note on confidentiality

SOME OF THE PEOPLE you will encounter in this book have not been anonymised and no details of their stories have been changed. Others have been anonymised to greater or lesser degrees. Sometimes a name change was all that was requested. Elsewhere, I've altered locations, dates and other identifying details. These decisions were made by the people whose stories I recount. – NF

The Language of Madness
(and the beginning of our conversation)

I REMEMBER THE FIRST TIME that I forcibly medicated a person against his will. It was thirteen years ago, not long after I'd qualified as a mental health nurse, and I had started my career working on a psychiatric ward providing assessment and treatment for adults in acute phases of serious mental illness.

There was a patient (or service user or client or son or brother or friend, depending on who you ask) whom I'll call Amit. Amit had been refusing any medication for nearly three weeks and with good reason. The medicine we were offering him contained a poison. It had been prescribed by a doctor who wished to harm him. In fact, this doctor – a consultant psychiatrist – had been struck off the medical register for his abuse of Amit during previous admissions and so was now working illegally on the ward. Many of the nursing staff knew this, and were in on it.

During morning medication round, Amit stood in the doorway of the ward clinic, watching me closely. He watched the movement of my hands over the drugs trolley as I secretly replaced his regular tablets with harmful ones.

He was wearing the same clothes that he'd slept in and a pair of old trainers, one with a huge split down the side. Another patient (or colleague or mother or teacher or daughter) had recently complained about Amit's smell. Whenever he sat in the TV lounge, she said, it made her feel physically sick. The problem was that Amit knew the water supply to his room was deliberately contaminated and so hadn't washed since he was admitted. I would try to talk to him about that again later – to find the right words – but for now, at least, the medication was the priority.

I double-checked the dose on his chart, put two tablets into a clear plastic pot and held it out for him to take.

He stared at it. We both did. I tried some words of reassurance. 'I know you're finding it hard to trust us at the moment, Amit. I do understand that. We think that's all a part of you being unwell again.'

He knew I was lying.

'I'll take them in my room,' he said.

I knew he was lying.

'You know it doesn't work that way. I'm sorry, but I need to see you take them.'

He cautiously reached out and took the pot from me. He prodded at the tablets inside. His fingers were stained dark yellow from tobacco. 'Nah. You're all right,' he said at last, placing the pot on top of the drugs trolley and backing out of the clinic, watching me the whole time. As he disappeared down the long corridor towards his bedroom, I wrote an 'R' for 'Refused' on his medication chart. Of course he refused. Why wouldn't he refuse? If I were in his position, I know I would.

But I don't know if I would refuse with the same dignity he showed when later that afternoon the C & R team entered his bedroom.

C & R. Control and Restraint. The legal (if controversial) techniques that mental health nurses are trained in to render a person unable to fight back. In subsequent years, this training would be rebranded as Prevention and Management of Violence and Aggression, which is reasonable if a person is smashing up the ward or threatening to hurt someone, but at times like this, for my money, the first description felt more honest.

It had been decided in a team meeting led by the consultant

psychiatrist that this was the last day Amit could refuse oral medication before we would use an injectable form. In the parlance of psychiatry: his mental state was deteriorating daily; he was well known to mental health services; and this was a typical presentation and pattern of his illness. If we could get him back on a stable dose of medication he'd likely respond well.

Amit was sitting on his bed, smoking and tuning through the static on a portable radio. He was talking to somebody that none of us could see. He looked up. There were five of us.

'Do I have to beg you?' he asked.

A colleague of mine explained his options, such as they were. But that's the bit that stayed with me. *Do I have to beg you?* It's why I struggled to keep my hands from shaking as he was eventually held down on his bed and I administered the injection. He didn't put up a fight. We weren't preventing and managing violence and aggression. From Amit's perspective, I don't doubt we were perpetrating it. In that moment, however good my intentions, I was knowingly participating in his suffering.

It was around this time that I began to write a novel. I was living in a small shared flat in inner-city Bristol, and between shifts on the ward I would sit for long hours at my desk – or more often pace the floorboards in the hope that the physical movement of my body might somehow dislodge some inspiration from whatever stone in my brain it was hiding beneath.

I was imagining the life of a young man who was suffering from the symptoms of a strange and commonly misunderstood illness (or disease or condition or trauma or phenomenon or curse or gift, depending on who you ask), and also the lives of this man's family and friends. This was a work of fiction but it was fiction that drew upon my very real feelings about working in mental healthcare, as well as many of my personal childhood experiences. I reckon that's where imagination comes from. Whether consciously or unconsciously, we dig up memories of our experiences – what we've *seen* and *done* and *read* and *felt* and *hoped* and *fucked up* and *desired* and *regretted* and all the rest of it – and then we reshape them a bit here, a bit there, until they resemble something entirely new. For the protagonist in my novel, though, experience and imagination had become inseparably tangled so that he no longer knew what was real and what was happening only inside his head. For me, understanding and responding to what this character was going through was principally an imaginative exercise. Or put another way: an act of empathy.

This is something that writing a novel (and reading one) and mental healthcare have in common. To do each of them well requires bucketloads of empathy; of striving to understand and share the feelings of other people. Of course, as an author of fiction, I was also responsible for *creating* the very problems that I then had to empathise with. Though, thinking about Amit, I probably did that as a nurse quite often too.

So my protagonist was having a hard time.

I decided not to diagnose him in the novel, but if I had, I'd have probably landed on schizophrenia.

Schizophrenia

What a word, huh?

I wonder if you might consider trying something for me? Say the word 'schizophrenia' out loud a few times. Not beneath your breath. Really say it. Say it loud enough that you feel self-conscious;

that you worry someone will hear. Say it loud enough that some-one might hear.

Feel the shape of it. Stay with it. Think about what that word evokes in you. What thoughts does it arrive with? What feelings?

Okay. That's the interactive part of this book over with. I promise I'll just let you read now. But please remember this as you do so: whole lives have disappeared beneath that word.

Schizophrenia is derived from the Greek *skhizein*, 'to split', and *phrēn*, 'mind'. Small wonder then that the perception of a divided person with two or more distinct personalities has endured so immutably in the public imagination. It's utter non-sense though.

Let's be clear about this from the start: *schizophrenia does not mean split personality*. Neither does it mean multiple personality. But declaring what it isn't is a good deal easier than asserting what it is.

There's credible and often heated debate across the fields of psychiatry, psychology, genetics, neuroscience and various mental health charities and campaign groups over everything from causes and risk factors to categorisation and treatments, and indeed as to whether the whole concept of the diagnosis has outlasted its use-fulness (if it ever was useful) and should be rebuilt from scratch or abandoned entirely.

If we tentatively take a seat in this debate the first thing that will become clear is that there is no uncontroversial language when talking about mental illness – and that includes the phrase 'mental illness'.

On the whole, the controversy around a term tends to relate to how medical it feels. Take the collective noun for people accessing mental health services. It was during my own nursing training that the word 'patient' fell almost entirely out of favour and we were encouraged instead to adopt 'service user' – to the confusion of many service users, granted.

In fact, the term had been a long time coming. It was the fruit of decades of campaigning by people who had themselves been 'patients' within the psychiatric system and who roundly rejected the medical connotations of the term: that it implies a doctor-knows-best passivity, compounding feelings of disempowerment. The term 'service user' was preferred because it defines a group by precisely that – its *use of services*, rather than by a sick role.

So already we can see the beginnings of an ideological split. If you're a user of mental health services and believe that your distressing thoughts and feelings are an illness, presumably located within your brain, and essentially the same as any physical illness, then you might well prefer to think of yourself as a patient. After all, if you're the same as those patients receiving care for broken bones and pneumonia and cancer and diabetes and chest infections then why should you be called something different?

However, if you're of the view – shared by many people, including many mental health professionals – that even the most alarming of your thoughts, and the most extreme changes in your moods, and your most uncharacteristic behaviours are not symptomatic of illness so much as a natural response to undischarged trauma or painful life events, then to see this wrapped up in the medical language of diagnosis that inevitably begins with you being declared a 'patient' might feel seriously problematic.

'Service user' was generally considered the more neutral term and so gained traction. But what about people like Amit? People who are detained in hospitals and medicated against their will? Does the collective noun of service user really cut it for them? Can we in all conscience say they are *using* mental health services?

Probably not.

Today there's a growing minority of people who eschew both terms and collectively self-identify as 'survivors', while the Council of the Royal College of Psychiatrists recently recommitted to 'patient'. And if all this sounds complicated and fraught with politics it's because it absolutely is. We've barely scratched the surface.[1]

It might be tempting to roll our eyes at this point.

To quote the protagonist of my novel, upon him hearing the term 'service user' for the first time:

> They have a bunch of names for us. Service Users must be the latest. I think there must be people who get paid to decide this shit.
>
> I thought about Steve. He's definitely the sort to say Service User. He'd say it like he deserved a knighthood for being all sensitive and empowering.[2]

(Steve, incidentally, is a mental health worker inspired by what I felt to be my own worst professional traits.)

I offer the quote because I think it's no bad thing to uphold a little cynicism. As with any impassioned debate, there are almost certainly elements of self-interest and prejudice on all sides. That said, I also believe it would be a grave mistake to dismiss any of this as unimportant. Yes, it's a dispute about language, but in the mad, mad world of mental healthcare *language is everything*. A simple truth, which we will confront in more detail later, is that the overwhelming majority of psychiatric diagnoses aren't arrived at by looking at blood tests or brain scans or anything of the sort. Rather, it is the *words* people say – or do not say – as interpreted by professionals, that as much as anything else will determine a diagnosis.

And the language of diagnosis, for better or worse, has the power to profoundly alter people's lives.

This brings us back to the word we were speaking out loud a few moments ago. And if something as seemingly innocuous as a simple word like 'patient' is the subject of such controversy, we can now begin to imagine the dark storms of debate swirling around the truly immense subject of 'schizophrenia'.

It is with this in mind that I want to make a commitment. From this paragraph forth the terminology in this book will either directly reflect that used by the people I meet (or whose writings I quote from) or else will strive to acknowledge that the most commonly used terms, as adopted largely from the world of medicine, represent only one way of thinking. To this end, *schizophrenia* will become *so-called schizophrenia* and a *mental illness*, a *so-called mental illness*. Or else I will use inverted commas or some other indicator to keep us mindful that there exist alternative narratives.

The novelist in me is cringing at the unwieldiness of this (while some other part of me doesn't especially enjoy being perched on this decidedly splintery fence), but I hope it will be seen for what it is: a genuine attempt to be respectful to both those who find comfort in the language of medicine and those who have been injured by it.

Okay. Let's try it out.

The controversies surrounding so-called schizophrenia are as old as the 'illness' itself.

There. That wasn't so difficult.

Now, as to precisely how old so-called schizophrenia is, needless to say, there's some debate.

On the whole, its discovery – or invention – is credited to the German psychiatrist Emil Kraepelin (1856–1926). He was the first physician to describe a 'precocious madness' that he observed in psychiatric patients and incorrectly hypothesised to be an early onset brain disease causing cognitive disintegration. He named this 'dementia praecox'. Then, during a lecture in Berlin on 24 April 1908, Kraepelin's contemporary Eugen Bleuler (1857–1939) made the successful case for a rebrand: 'schizophrenia' was born.

What Kraepelin and Bleuler could not have anticipated was that their mysterious new disorder with its exotic-sounding name would in time come to be seen as the very heartland of psychiatry; the condition that defines the discipline.[3] Such is the seriousness and complexity of the disorder that to understand it, so this theory goes, is to understand mental health.

It is for precisely this reason that this book will use the diagnosis of 'schizophrenia' as the landscape from which to explore broader notions of health, suffering and the whole curious absurdity of being human. This terrain is far from peaceful. The heartland is the bloody battleground upon which the fiercest ideological disputes about madness and its meanings are fought.[*]

Believe me when I tell you that these disputes are *fierce*. Many of the issues we will cover in this book are also right at this moment being debated by leading mental health clinicians and academics, and if you happen to take a cursory look on social media to find these debates you won't have to scroll for very long before you encounter what *Mental Health Today* calls a 'bitter adversarial dynamic'.[4] Curiously, a great deal of this acrimony exists between two professional guilds that work closely alongside each other and that many people assume are one and the same thing. I'm talking here about the distinct but related disciplines of *psychiatry* and *psychology*.

---

[*] I first read about schizophrenia being referred to as the heartland in *The British Journal of Psychiatry*. It's an emotive, strangely territorial description. It's not a phrase used today, but it remains apt to describe what is a highly emotive and proprietorial debate.

The lexicon of mental healthcare involves a lot of these 'psych' words. It's a prefix that occurs in this book 343 times.* These words will, at least at first glance, feel familiar to most readers. They've found their way into common parlance through popular culture. However, they're often misused and confused. And that's for the very good reason that they're confusing.

So let's spend a moment getting to grips with a few of them.

Psychology

Psychology is the broadest of all the 'psych' words that appear in these pages. It is the scientific and social study of all aspects of our mental and behavioural lives. It's a discipline of enormous scope and diversity (if you're thinking or feeling it, psychology has a theory about it).

Clinical psychology is one of many specialisms within this field and is the one that is most pertinent to us here. It focuses on understanding, preventing and treating mental distress and dysfunction – often framed as 'mental illness'. *Clinical psychologists* must do an undergraduate degree in psychology and a further three-year postgraduate training at doctoral level.

The main method of treatment employed by psychologists is called *psychotherapy* (yet another 'psych-' word). Sometimes we simply call this 'talking therapy'. There are countless iterations of talking therapies, ranging from psychoanalysis, as developed by Sigmund Freud in the late 1800s, to the currently more fashionable mindfulness-based therapies and Cognitive Behavioural Therapy (CBT).

---

* To put that in perspective, it's 340 times more often than Ant McPartlin and Declan Donnelly implored us to watch them 'wreck the mic – psyche!' in their 1994 debut studio album *Psyche*.

Many of the professionals that we will hear from in this book are clinical psychologists.

Psychiatry

In contrast to psychology, *psychiatry* is a medical profession. *Psychiatrists* are medical doctors who do the usual five-year training at medical school before going on to specialise in mental health.

They are similarly concerned with mental distress, though they often place a greater emphasis on biological causes and medical treatments. In other words, they frame mental illness – at least in part – as the consequence of chemical imbalances within the brain, which other chemicals might be used to redress. Psychiatrists (unlike clinical psychologists) will therefore frequently prescribe medication, although it's important to add that many psychiatrists offer talking therapies too.

In the UK, psychiatrists are also charged with making more decisions regarding the detention and enforced treatment of people under the Mental Health Act.

In the NHS – and in most western healthcare systems – it is a biomedical approach, as most closely associated with psychiatry, that has become the dominant paradigm for conceptualising and treating serious mental distress.

This has not always been the case. In our long history of trying to get to grips with human madness, different ideologies have enjoyed their moment in the sun. Go back far enough and we inevitably encounter demons and spirits (which still feature in some cultures, of course).

Even as recently as the twentieth century, the newly conceived profession of psychiatry wasn't overly concerned with biological mechanisms.* Or rather, after an initial and ultimately fruitless effort to find madness spelled out on the physical matter of the brain, it turned its attention instead to psychoanalysis, and for many years a person's life history and childhood were deemed to be most significant when trying to understand and treat them.

It was only in the decades after the Second World War, crucially coinciding with the invention of new medications and the publication of a now legendary classification system for mental disorders (more on these things later), that modern psychiatry nailed its colours to the mast as a truly medical discipline, in the sense that we understand the term today.

Many people – including numerous psychiatrists, other health professionals and people who use psychiatric services – believe that this represents good progress and is a clear sign that we're heading in the right direction.

Many other people – including numerous psychiatrists, other health professionals and people who use psychiatric services – are profoundly critical of this, and fear we're doing more harm than good.

Psychosis

Of all the 'psych-' words in this book, the one most loaded with popular misconceptions is *psychosis*. It's an important one for us, not least because it's generally considered to be a defining feature of so-called schizophrenia.

---

* Psychiatry was officially created in 1808 when the German physician Johann Christian Reil had the neat idea of joining together the Greek terms *psyche*, meaning 'soul' or 'spirit' (and so casting Ant and Dec's later work into its truly philosophical context), and –*iatry*, meaning 'medical treatment'.

I remember the first time that I encountered this word in a clinical setting.

I was nineteen years old and was beginning my career in mental health as a health care assistant, providing short-term cover for wards with staff shortages. HCAs are often highly skilled and well-trained members of a hospital workforce. I was not. My interview for the job, such as it was, can't have lasted more than ten minutes and was mostly concerned with my availability. My point is that I knew nothing. I remember arriving for my first shift. It was at a psychiatric hospital on the outskirts of Bristol, in the green and leafy grounds of an old Victorian workhouse and lunatic asylum. A crackly intercom on the locked front door instructed me to head to the nursing office. I hesitated. With all the usual anxieties that come with starting any new job there was something else in the mix. Until this point my only real experience of so-called serious mental illness had come from the stuff I'd discovered second-hand, from books, films, TV and the tabloid newspapers that my parents read throughout my childhood. My head was filled with precon-ceptions and misconceptions about mental institutions, asylums, madhouses and the kinds of people in them.

I feverishly scribbled down notes as, one by one, nurses from the previous shift came into a cluttered office to hand over relevant details about the patients they'd been working with, and what needed to be done during the rest of the day. I'd never written the word 'psychotic' before. I wasn't even sure how to spell it. But now I was writing it over and over. I didn't know what it meant, but it came with a feeling attached – a physical feeling, a perceptible tightening in my chest.

During that first shift, I spent most of my time sitting in a dreary smoking room, drinking tea with 'psychotic people', and wonder-ing what I was meant to say. I remember meeting a woman who was recovering from a first episode of what may have been 'bipolar disorder' – she was getting better, but she was terribly shaken. She took a long drag of her cigarette and told me that before she came onto the ward she hadn't known such places really existed.[5]

Me neither, I thought.

Though not an especially precise term, at its broadest and most simplistic psychosis describes the phenomenon of a person losing contact with reality – or, at any rate, losing contact with what most other people *perceive* as reality.

It's not considered to be an illness or disease in and of itself, though it can certainly be symptomatic of disease. It's a typical feature in most forms of dementia, for instance.

Many of us will experience psychosis at some point in our lives; we may even actively pursue it. It's the desired effect of numerous recreational drugs. If you try LSD and it doesn't radically distort your experience of reality, then I suggest you find a new dealer.

Importantly, what we call psychosis can also be a response to extreme stress or trauma. As we'll revisit later, for many people it might best be understood as a kind of psychological adaptation, a coping strategy gone awry or a form of storytelling carried out within the mind as a response to unbearably painful life events. Whatever its cause, psychosis is commonly experienced through *hallucinations* and *delusions*. Hallucination is the medical name given to false sensory experiences, such as hearing voices or seeing things that other people can't. Delusions are usually false and bizarre beliefs that are held with conviction and are unresponsive to evidence proving them to be wrong. Amit's belief that we were contaminating the water supply to his bedroom could be described as a delusion. It might also be described as an understandable response to what was happening to him.

Most people who are diagnosed as having schizophrenia experience this kind of detachment from reality. Often – though not always – this is deeply distressing and can lead to strange behaviours as the person tries to navigate and survive in their altered, hostile world.

Psychosis may be a major feature of so-called schizophrenia, but it's by no means the whole picture.

Other symptoms can include: a disintegration in the process of thinking; disorganised speech; disorganised behaviour; flattened or incongruous emotional responses; impaired attention and significant social withdrawal.

These are often sub-categorised (a little confusingly) into *positive* and *negative* symptoms. In this case positive doesn't signify a symptom being beneficial or good, but rather that it's an addition to a person's consciousness. Hallucinations and delusions are therefore positive symptoms, whereas social withdrawal, avolition (a lack of motivation to accomplish purposeful, even pleasurable tasks) and poverty of speech are negative symptoms, as they each represent something that has been lost.

In a popular TED talk, Professor Elyn Saks, an expert in mental health who herself lives with a schizophrenia diagnosis, asserts: 'The schizophrenic mind is not split but shattered.'[6] It's also a surprisingly common phenomenon. A statistic bandied around for years is that worldwide it affects around one in every hundred people, though this distribution is far from even.[7] The rates of psychotic disorders, including so-called schizophrenia, are higher in men than women. They are also higher in younger age groups, and in racial and ethnic minorities. And there's huge variation, not only by person but by place. More on that later.

———

I mentioned that not long after I'd finished my training and began working as a registered mental health nurse, I also started to try to write a novel. There's a nice Peter Cook quote that pretty much sums up my experience of this: 'I met a man at a party. He said, "I'm writing a novel." I said, "Oh really? Neither am I."'

Yet a mere nine years after I'd first sat in front of my computer to stare hopelessly at a blank page, my novel was – by some miracle – finished and on the shelves.* A lot can happen in nine years. I'd left frontline nursing to work in mental health research at the University of Bristol. I'd also had a baby daughter, got married, and was wondering whether I should maybe try and write another book one day and if my own mental health would survive it. Then the emails arrived through the contact page of my shiny new author website.

They were from people I'd never met but who had read my fictional account of a young man with 'schizophrenia' and had taken the time to reach out and share their own stories – true stories – sometimes because they were similar; sometimes because they were wholly different.

And this conversation grew as I continued to meet more people through my work writing and speaking about mental health.

Many of the stories told to me were upsetting, others hopeful. Rarely did they have the kind of neatly conceived beginning, middle and end that as a novelist I had the luxury to craft. A truth about the strange phenomenon we call mental illness is that it's messy and chaotic; it can be extremely difficult to make sense of, but that

---

* So yes, needless to say, I found writing a novel really, really, really difficult and frequently responded to this by not writing it. This is a well-established technique for the first-time novelist and one that I wholeheartedly endorse.

doesn't mean we shouldn't try. There's a fragility to the mental health of everyone. It serves us all to be part of the conversation.

That's what this book is: a part of the conversation.

I'd like to introduce you to some people that I've been fortunate enough to meet. I'm going to tell you their stories and after each story I'll reflect a little on what it might teach us and what questions it raises.

We will consider such topics as stigma (and why the current conversations around stigma could be missing the point); diagnosis (and why psychiatric diagnostics is on seriously shaky ground); the causes of 'mental illness' (and why nobody can say with absolute certainty what makes any given individual become 'unwell'); delusions and hallucinations (and how these are a part of all of our lives, all of the time); and psychiatric medication (including the things that 'patient information leaflets' don't tell us).

In debates characterised by increasingly polarised positions, we'll attempt the more revolutionary approach of trying to keep an open mind.

In this way, I hope that we'll untangle a few of the more pernicious myths and stereotypes that the very word 'schizophrenia' so stubbornly evokes, and also that we'll arrive at some clarity about our own mental wellbeing and that of others.

The Mad Hatter (the one from *Batman*, not *Alice's Adventures in Wonderland*) once explained that trying to understand madness with logic is 'not unlike searching for darkness with a torch'.[8] Putting aside that he was an evil supervillain, and maybe not the best exemplar of mental health portrayals in fiction, he still had a point. The logic of scientific research – which will certainly form a part of this book – can only take us so far. There is another part of the thing we call 'mental illness' that will for ever exist beyond the reach of statistical analysis, probabilities and distribution curves, or the otherworldly pictures of neurochemical imaging.

It is the person. It is their story.

Sitting in that hospital smoking room during my first shift as a care assistant, I was too nervous to open my mouth. I had no idea what to say, which by chance meant I probably did the best thing. I listened. It's not always possible to find the right words but we can still be part of the conversation. We can walk with people for a bit, sit with them, hear them.

THE JOURNALIST

The fugitive

UPON BEING NAMED BRITAIN'S most wanted criminal, twenty-nine-year-old Molly went to her local supermarket, where she bought a bottle of bleach to drink.

She stopped briefly to look at the rack of newspapers and her worst fears were confirmed. The *Daily Mirror* – a newspaper she had previously contributed articles to – had launched a hate campaign against her. The other papers each carried headlines and stories pertaining to her crimes. These included the false imprisonment and sexual assault of a friend she knew from her university days; her suspected role in the unsolved murder of a young man at a London squat party; and her involvement in a conspiracy to detonate a bomb in Canary Wharf shortly after 9/11. There were other crimes, too numerous for Molly to recall. Her double life was coming to an end. The police were closing in. Helicopters circled the night sky.

Clutching her bottle of bleach, Molly hurried back home. These streets were unfamiliar. Over the past ten years, Molly had moved around a lot, rarely staying at a job or flat for more than a few months. Mostly she moved around London, and a couple of times to New York. Recently she'd lived and worked in the south of England as a university lecturer. That's where things really started to unravel, but there was no point thinking about that any more. Right now she was in a rundown neighbourhood of inner-city Birmingham, avoiding eye contact with everyone she passed, convinced they knew exactly who she was and exactly what she had done. More strangely: these people also knew what she was about to do. And they were pleased about it. *Thank God she's finally going to die.*

Back at her flat, Molly took a mug from the shared kitchen and shut herself in her bedroom.

She filled the mug with bleach, and drank it.

Seven years later she can still taste it: the thickness, the bitterness.

We are chatting together in Molly's immaculate, art-filled living room at her home in Derby – a vintage suitcase is open on the carpet between us, spilling out clippings of her many articles and editorials for national tabloids, glossy fashion mags, obscure low-res fanzines and serious scientific newsletters.

She struggles not to gag at the memory. 'It's just hard,' she explains. 'Thinking about that horrible room, and my flatmates not knowing what was going on. My family so unsupportive.'

The Waltons and the Cluster Fuck

Molly grew up in Castleton, a picturesque village at the edge of the Hope Valley in the Derbyshire Peak District. Her mum was a housewife; her dad sold antiques. She describes her early years as idyllic – at least, that's how her mum liked to think of them. She would make clothes for Molly and her younger sister. She made their school uniforms. She even made the jam that went in the brown bread sandwiches in their lunch boxes. Molly hints at there being an affected quality to all this: 'I think Mum liked to believe we were the Waltons.' Her parents had grown up poor on council estates but money was no longer a problem. Her dad's business was doing extremely well. They were getting wealthy under Thatcher, rapidly climbing the socio-economic ladder. I ask Molly if she considers her upbringing to have been typically middle-class, but she shakes her head and settles on 'nouveau riche'.

She recalls that at eight years old, prior to starting middle school, she begged to be sent to a private school. She was unusually driven and can distinctly recall speaking with a friend's parents in the village and them impressing upon her how important it was to get the best possible start in life. In the event, Molly was sent to the local state school and her dad bought a new BMW. Many years later, as part of something Molly calls 'Project Dad' she would find out exactly the cost of that BMW and the cost of the tuition fees.

Nevertheless, Molly thrived at school. She was pretty, popular and ambitious. She became a member of the Press Pack for BBC *Newsround* and used to write plays and radio shows that she'd rehearse and perform with her friends. She was also eccentric. 'I used to make things up,' she tells me. 'I'd go to the headmaster and say things like, "Did you know it's National Pizza Day today?" and try to get him to order pizzas.' She started her own gym class in the school gym and persuaded other children to sign up. She was constantly dreaming up elaborate schemes, and in telling me about them she borrows a term straight out of a psychiatric textbook: *flight of ideas*. It's a phrase commonly associated with the so-called manic disorders such as bipolar, and describes a rapid flow of thought with abrupt changes from one idea to the next.

It's also – of course – a perfectly normal characteristic of an energetic and intellectually curious child. I pause on it only because of what Molly says next: 'I was never bullied for being different. But I *was* different.'

'Your dad's done something terrible,' Molly's mum told her. 'It's not your fault.'

Molly was eleven years old and was hiding in the loo. She'd been listening to her mum screaming at her dad to leave them alone. 'The children are asleep, the children are asleep!'

He was smashing down the front door.

The terrible thing, according to Molly's mum, was that her dad was having an affair. What followed was a violent and intensely acrimonious breakdown of their marriage, with Molly and her younger sister caught in the middle. Her sister dealt with the trauma by closing down, shutting herself away in her room and not talking to anyone.

It was Molly whom their mum frequently confided in. She began drinking heavily and would drunkenly wake Molly up late at night, sit on her bed and talk about what a bastard her dad was. It was a horrible time. The end of the Waltons and the start of what Molly now calls the Cluster Fuck.

No longer getting the right kind of love at home, she began acting out at school. By age twelve she was frequently bunking off, heading out into the countryside with friends and smoking weed or getting plastered on White Lightning until she was sick. By fourteen or fifteen she had discovered clubbing and harder drugs. She started taking a lot of speed (£5 wraps of 'Pink Champagne' that she'd bomb or snort). Molly was losing her way in life. On one occasion she walked out of a drama class to smoke in the toilets and tried to start a fire. The toilet roll was hanging in a plastic shell and she set it alight. She was bored, angsty and couldn't give a fuck. Gone were her childhood ambitions. When she eventually left school with four Cs at GCSE, her only plan was to get a job as a cleaner, buy nice dresses and go clubbing.

I wonder what her parents made of all this? Molly is succinct: 'Mum tried her best, but you can't bring up young children when you're drunk.'

Her dad, now living with his new girlfriend, stepped up. In a small twist of irony, he bribed Molly to stay in education with the promise of buying her a new car – a black Fiat Uno with alloy wheels. She enrolled at a local college to do a BTEC in fashion design. She picked it because she thought it'd be a doss. It turned out she had a talent for it. Yet her mental state remained, in her words, on a knife edge. She recalls a day at college, an illustration lesson. She'd just returned to class from a cigarette break, took her seat, and fell to pieces. Huge, heaving, noisy sobs for what might have been half an hour, with nobody able to console her. In the end the tutor had no choice but to send her home. To this day, Molly has no idea what came over her. It was also at college that, following a break-up with a boyfriend, Molly began abusing laxatives, becoming what she calls a 'functioning bulimic'.

For all this, she did well on the course, and a couple of years later successfully applied to study fashion at Middlesex University, attending the interview wearing a dress she'd made herself. She moved to London, into a small council flat in Bethnal Green. This flat was done out in a sixties style, complete with orange laminate surfaces. Molly loved it. She bought vintage peacock chairs, a Tretchikoff print to hang on the wall. She liked her flatmate, liked the course. She was making a home. She'd finally pulled through the Cluster Fuck. Then things took a turn for the worse.

Rebirthing

It's a bit blurry but it went something like this. Molly was in the Student Union bar and wasn't feeling too great. She was worried about her mum's drinking, and that since moving to London she wasn't there to help her. She was worried that her dad didn't help either. She was worried that she wasn't as thin as the other girls on her course. She was worried that her flatmate wanted them to move out of their place in Bethnal Green and find somewhere bigger with a third person. She was worried about why this worried her so much, and was feeling confused about her sexuality. She must have looked distressed, because someone approached to offer comfort.

Molly knew this girl a little from the course. She was from South Korea, and to Molly she was an impressive figure: worldly and composed. Molly felt touched that she was even giving her the time of day – asking what was wrong, offering encouragement. She had already begun to think of her as an angel when the girl said, 'You will see the light.'

For the next week Molly ate nothing but Farley's Rusks. She didn't tell anyone what she was doing but she knew instinctively that to 'see the light' she would need to 'rebirth herself' – a process that became tangled up in her already complicated relationship with food. By eating the rusks she would get back in touch with her inner child. Nothing happened though, so Molly realised she needed to up her game. If she stopped eating altogether she would move into an altered consciousness and find God there. For the next seven months she ate only to survive. Half a Ryvita for breakfast, and a low-calorie soup with half a boiled onion later in the day. It was still too much so she returned to abusing laxatives, eating up to two whole packets at a time. She became skeletally thin, stopped menstruating and constantly came down with viruses and infections. Then one night Molly went out clubbing with friends and took some ecstasy. She stepped outside for a cigarette and whatever she said to the bouncer made him concerned enough that he told her she needed to find her friends and go home. She only remembers a powerful sense of being completely lost in the world. The next day, she woke up certain that she had committed a terrible crime, and that the police were coming to get her.

Sniff, sniff

And so began Molly's life as a fugitive. It was also around this time that she started working for a national broadsheet newspaper.

This was her second year of university and she had arranged a placement with the paper's fashion desk. It was fairly menial work, mostly sorting clothes for photoshoots, then packing them away to return to the suppliers. Other work experience students didn't want to do that sort of thing; they wanted to be writing the stories. But Molly was fine with it. By this time she hoped to become a fashion assistant, and this seemed as good a way in as any. After the two-week placement, the paper offered to keep her on for a day a week. She says she was their 'Girl Friday'. In return for her services they paid for her weekly travelcard.

Her colleagues liked her. She worked hard and was personable. She was also stylish, attractive, thin as a rake, and more than prepared to party hard. She was a natural fit for the world of fashion. 'Fashion has its own kind of bulimia,' she tells me. 'It latches on to anything young and new, then when you get older it regurgitates you.'

By this time she was living in a house in Homerton, East London, with a couple of third years. One evening Molly locked herself out – she was losing her keys and credit cards all the time. Both of her housemates were away, and so Molly waited in a local pub drinking pints of Guinness, which she considered a substitute for food. She drank a lot that night, then at closing time – upon being kicked out – she became horribly afraid. She stills feels some justification for this. The area was infamous at the time for its high crime rates, the so-called 'murder mile'. Molly smashed a kitchen window to get inside her house. When her housemate returned later and saw the damage, she screamed at Molly, 'So you're an alcoholic as well as an anorexic now.' She then burst into tears. It was the end of their friendship, and Molly felt forced to move out.

At the newspaper, though, she felt more accepted. She felt safe there. 'Even though they're a pool of sharks,' she laughs. Molly was promoted to the role of fashion assistant, supporting the deputy fashion editor. She was making this job her life and dropped out of university.

She had still received no professional input about her eating or any of her strange thoughts. Nobody in her life had suggested that she might need help. 'I wonder if it happened today if it would be different?' she considers. 'If people would be more supportive. But I didn't think to share my thoughts. I didn't think your thoughts could be unwell.' She did, however, decide that she ought to try to put on some weight. At its lowest, Molly's weight plummeted to little more than five stone. She was now up to around seven stone, but at five foot seven she knew she still needed to put on more. Her strategy was to smoke weed: 'To help relax at work and to get the munchies.' She bought some skunk at London Bridge and went back home to the flat in Catford where she was now lodging. Molly smoked the skunk in the back garden, then went inside and lay on her bed. That's when the people started watching her. Her friends and her colleagues. They could all see her and they all knew what she was doing in her bedroom.

And what was she doing?

'Blinking. They were watching my blinking. Should I blink? Should I keep my eyes open or close them? People were laughing at me, ridiculing me. My blinking was wrong.'

The next night she did it all over again.

Of course, Molly isn't the first person to have felt a bit strange after smoking strong cannabis. The problem was that increasingly strange things were starting to happen in her life even when she wasn't using drugs. It was around this time that she befriended a group of squatters and was going to squat parties. She lost her keys at one of these in Shoreditch, returning the next morning to get them. Her friends left her waiting at the door for the longest time, then when they eventually invited her in they showed her an art project that a couple of them were working on. Black-and-white photographs of people crying. One of them was of a man crying, curled up on the floor, naked. This made sense. It was because Molly had done something terrible at the party and the photo was her friends' way of telling her how she ought to be feeling.

It was also around this time, following a one-night stand with a guy she met at a gallery opening in Brick Lane, that Molly decided to get a coil fitted. Except this was no ordinary coil. She only realised as she walked away from the sexual health clinic that they had fitted a camera into her womb. This too made perfect sense. It was MI5's way of tracking her.

———

I want to check something with Molly at this point. It's occurred to me that these two beliefs have quite different qualities. On the one hand there is the abstract, almost dreamlike notion that the photograph of the crying man was a signpost to how she should be feeling. Then there is – to my mind, anyway – the markedly more concrete belief that her contraceptive coil was a piece of spy equipment, one that had been placed inside her by MI5 with the specific purpose of tracking her movements. There is nothing intangible about that. It's not a vague paranoia about what people might be thinking. The coil was in place. It was either an MI5 camera or it wasn't.

I pause on it because I want to understand the way these more bizarre beliefs take hold compared to her other beliefs.

We frequently challenge and doubt information that we receive from, let's call it, 'the real world'. For example, if we watch a reality TV show, we might decide that everything we are watching is entirely real and true to life, but equally we might be sceptical about certain elements, or indeed we might consider the whole thing to be contrived. Our understanding of the world is obviously informed by our experiences but we also have within us the faculty to doubt the veracity of these experiences, and to alter our beliefs in the wake of additional evidence. I'm trying to understand whether it was intrinsic to the nature of Molly's more unusual beliefs that they left no room for doubt.

It's a longwinded way of asking: How certain were you that your coil was an MI5 camera?

———

Molly lights a cigarette and thinks on this for a while. We've come out into her garden to drink tea and sit together in a small patch of spring sunshine. 'I can't have been that certain,' she concludes. 'Because if I was that certain I would have been more freaked out than I was. It kind of came in waves. I wasn't always thinking like that. It was like—' Molly stops and sniffs at the air. 'You know when you kind of sniff something in the air. It's like that. Like just getting a whiff of something. Except it's sniffing a thought.'

She gives an example of what she means. She recalls a walk to work one morning, to the newspaper offices, which at that time were in Canary Wharf. She passes a newsagent on the way and catches sight of a copy of the magazine *Sleazenation*. The headline is along the lines of: 'We need revolution!' It's enough to give Molly a whiff of something. She begins to think about the squatters that she's been hanging around with. Perhaps they aren't quite what they appear to be. They're all involved in the art world. The headline could be a message from them. This is shortly after 9/11 and it occurs to Molly that they're trying to get her to blow up Canary Wharf. They want a revolution and as a person who knows them but also works in the corporate world, she's the ideal target to plant a bomb. She gets to the office, opens her notepad, picks up her pen with the big feather on top and attempts to crack on with her to-do list – *get photographic film out of fridge, write captions for latest shoot, call in clothes for the next shoot, clean out storage cupboard* – all the while terrified that she's going to be forced to do something horrendous, something she knows she doesn't want to do.

I find Molly's capacity to have kept going through all of this, without any help from anyone, to be more than a little humbling. For the first time in our conversation, I find myself using a medical term. I say it's extraordinary that she was managing to hold her life together, more than hold it together, start to build a career, while 'clearly so psychotic'.

We fall into a brief silence. Then Molly says something that surprises me. 'It's good to hear that. Because I haven't really gone into much detail about this period. It's kind of off the radar when I talk to clinicians because I talk about my recent problems, so it's good to get clarity that clearly that's psychosis, because sometimes I still do think, you know, that I've done something.'

Unwell thoughts

After a year and a half working at the newspaper, Molly's relationship with her editor was breaking down. She was finding it increasingly difficult to concentrate, was making too many mistakes. She recalls being reprimanded because the shirts she brought in for a

Victorian photo shoot weren't Victorian enough. She recalls over-hearing her editor on the phone saying, 'I can't stand her any more.' Molly knew this comment was about her and so began planning her escape.

It was a beautiful sunny day when Molly climbed up a grassy hill in a park in South East London, to take in the view and sketch out her future.

She was now twenty-three years old. She opened up her notebook and began writing down her goals. Among them: 'Travel, volunteer for disadvantaged people, finish my degree and get a Master's.' Molly laughs. 'There were other stupid things too . . . get a Maltese terrier, marry a rapper.'

Music – and especially hip hop – was an important part of Molly's life, and a significant motivator in her decision to add 'live and work in New York' to her list. It was the place where so much of the music that she loved was made. It was also reassuringly far away. Three months after making her list, she was on the plane. I wonder if Molly was running towards something or running away? She concedes it was a bit of both. By this time she had received some counselling on the NHS for her eating disorder – though she had still not spoken about the many other strange fears that drifted heavily through her thoughts. She had come to realise that her issues around food were related to her mum's drinking and concluded it would be best not to settle down too close to home.

In New York, Molly found a cheap hostel in Spanish Harlem, which she mostly shared with out-of-work actors who put in shifts at Burger King between auditions and hoping for their lucky break.

Molly was unemployed. Prior to setting off she'd sent her CV to the editor of a fashion and lifestyle magazine but had received no reply. Now she emailed again: *I'm here!*

Looking back, she believes the editor felt guilty, took pity on this young kid who had come all the way from England. There were no positions at the magazine but the editor set Molly up with some office work at a photography agency.

That's when things started turning soft. Molly recalls an occasion with some colleagues. They were all about to get into the office elevator but Molly couldn't step through the doors. The floor of the elevator had become somehow soft like putty and she knew that if she stepped on it, she would sink right through. She held everyone back, terrified.

Later, everything became soft, herself included. She felt her body being stretched and twisted. Molly attributed this to a kind of spiritual experience, an alteration of her consciousness.

It was entirely more pedestrian concerns that would drive her back to the UK. Her salary was little more than $50 a week, she had maxed out her credit cards and now her work visa was set to expire, meaning if she stayed she'd be working illegally. She feared becoming stranded, unable to afford a flight home.

And so it was that a few months after arriving in New York, Molly found herself penniless and living back with her mum and sister in her childhood home.

The messages and symbols were now all around her.

A song on the radio – 'Sweet Dreams my LA Ex', by Rachel Stevens – was a message from the London squatters: 'Sweet dreams, you laxative abuser. You're going to prison.' An oblique phone call from a friend Molly knew from her partying days at university contained evidence that Molly had committed a sex crime against her. The friend never said this, and Molly had no recollection of the crime, but she became feverishly obsessed with the idea, ordering old bank statements to help piece together her movements from five years previously, and staying up late into the night looking at articles her various editors had written, searching for metaphors and hidden messages that might reveal both what she had done and who else knew about it.

Molly began to prepare for prison. She bought an outfit to wear in court. She grew her hair. If she could make herself look as young and pretty as possible nobody would believe she could have committed these crimes.

All the while, she continued working. She enrolled on an online feature-writing course. If the screen flickered it was because someone was hacking into her computer. To pay off her debts she took a job as a medical receptionist. One morning a contractor came in under the pretence of needing to fix the fax machine but secretly wired up spy equipment inside it. Molly became hysterical, breaking down in tears and insisting to her colleagues that she was being set up, that people were coming to get her. She was told to take the day off. Then she was sacked for gross misconduct.

It was around three o'clock in the morning when Molly's mum found her under the bed looking for surveillance equipment.

Unable to contain her fears any longer, Molly confided in her mum, who persuaded her to see a GP. In the waiting room was a small, high window with bars across it – a clear sign that if she told the doctor what was happening she would be locked up.

Defeated and with thoughts of ending her own life, Molly told him anyway. The doctor prescribed her a course of sleeping tablets and referred her for an assessment with a psychiatrist.

It's not such a big deal for Molly to talk about having a psychotic illness today. She's written extensively about her experiences across the national press and given many talks and lectures. Psychosis

isn't such a scary word for her. It can even be – at least to a degree
– a reassuring one.

Her first encounter with it was a different story.

Molly liked the psychiatrist. She remembers he talked openly
with her about 'false beliefs'. For the first time since the world
had turned against her, she considered the idea that a person's
thoughts could, in her words, 'become poorly'. Until now she had
always viewed her mind as a spiritual thing, but chatting with the
psychiatrist, she contemplated the notion that her thoughts were
somehow unwell.

The psychiatrist referred Molly to a specialist community team
and also prescribed her a medication, which he explained was to
help with her unusual thinking. He didn't, at this time, speculate
with Molly about any possible diagnosis. But the word 'psychotic'
did make its way into her medical notes – as Molly would discover
a couple of weeks later during a routine smear test.

Catching on fire

Molly was already feeling confused. The nurse who was carrying
out her smear test commented on her contraceptive coil, asking
how long it had been in place. Except Molly didn't have a coil. She
was certain she didn't. She would have remembered.

She argued this to the nurse, who in turn argued that Molly
definitely did have one – she knew, because she was looking at it.

This was the same coil that a couple of years previously Molly
believed had been fitted by MI5. Now she had no recollection of its
existence. The nurse pulled up Molly's medical notes on the computer. Molly looked at the screen and that's when she saw it.

'Am I psychotic?' she asked.

The nurse glanced at the notes. 'It would appear so.'

Recalling the moment, Molly likens it to noticing that an item of her clothing had caught on fire. 'It was like there was something dangerous on me,' she explains. 'I'd read in the paper about people with psychosis having children and murdering them. That was the main story that I could think of. And I just thought, if I have kids I might murder them. Or if I told people the truth about my illness they would be terrified of me. And it just felt like having some kind of item of clothing that you're wearing on fire. I was scared. I thought that maybe I was actually dangerous.'[1]

She wasn't the only one with these fears. The hardest thing for Molly during this time was that her sister and mum seemed more afraid than they were concerned for her. She recalls her sister calling her a 'freak'. Her mum kicked her out of the family home. After a short while she was invited back, but Molly felt unwanted. On reflection she knows that her family simply had the same views and misconceptions that she herself held.

She returns to the phrase that she first used when describing her family: nouveau riche. 'We had a big house,' she tells me. 'But we didn't have any cultural capital or education. My mum wasn't about to go and research what psychosis was on the internet or read a book about it. It was more like: we know about this and we *know* that it's dangerous.'

(Mild) schizophrenia

Now taking a low dose of antipsychotic medication, Molly began to challenge some of her assumptions. Perhaps she wasn't a sex offender or a terrorist or a murderer. Her activities were not being monitored by MI5. She was sleeping better at night.

But her relationship with her mum and sister remained deeply fraught. She moved back to New York for a short while before returning to London, where she continued to move between jobs and homes at a dizzying rate – something she says is the nature of the beast.

The beast being 'schizophrenia'.

It was a psychiatrist Molly saw in London who finally made the diagnosis. He prefixed it with 'mild'. Though still feeling persecuted and bullied, she had by now successfully completed a foundation degree in journalism at the London College of Communication. She was being paid to write freelance articles. She was paying her rent. She was also in a relationship, although her partner at this time struggled to accept her diagnosis and was frustrated by how withdrawn Molly had become. She rarely went out and would spend long evenings at home, researching schizophrenia online.

She secretly took to Gumtree and typed: 'I've got schizophrenia. Does anyone else have it? Will you talk to me?'

She was shocked and saddened by some of the stories that came her way: stories of horrific abuse, rape, child sex abuse. 'It was really putting my story into perspective,' she tells me. She remembers once going to see her psychiatrist and there was a man in the reception area. 'His face was covered in cigarette burns,' she says. 'He was pacing up and down in this really small space and burning his face over and over with a cigarette. And there I was feeling a bit worried about being bullied at work and that *was* mild. In the grand scheme of things.'

In part to support a friend who suffered from obsessive–compulsive disorder, Molly found an informal mental health support group and frequently met up with them in a cafe in Queen's Park. She made a good group of friends there. She was getting interesting freelance work: blogging for a couple of national newspapers and working on a project with Channel 4. She wrote occasional pieces about living with her illness, too. She met a new boyfriend, fell in love, went travelling. For a period of several years Molly's life was back on track. She began reading R. D. Laing, traditional psychiatry's most famous and iconic critic, and encouraged by a friend from the cafe group, she decided to wean herself off medication.

She was feeling great. Better than great. She started to feel what she describes as 'the opposite of paranoia'. Everything in the world was working to help her. She might be a wizard of some kind, a shaman, have special powers. She broke up with her boyfriend but they remained close, and this too felt like it was the best thing that had ever happened to her.

Then at age twenty-nine, Molly was considering her career options. A position came up for a lecturer in fashion journalism. It would mean another move, this time to the south coast. At the interview Molly gave a presentation on how she was 'a fashion writer but actually a charlatan' on account of the fact that even a cover story she had written for *Nylon* magazine in the US only earned her $30. She was motivated by giving an honest account of the struggles of freelancing to the students.

Her interviewers loved it. She got the job.

Within a couple of months, things were going awry. A disgruntled student had found an online article that Molly had written for the *Mirror* about her experience of living with psychosis. It was spread around quickly on Facebook. Now everyone was reading it.

'It got completely ridiculed,' Molly tells me. 'I was seen as a joke.'

She'd already been struggling with certain aspects of the job, not least her Tuesday morning lectures where she would be faced with 140 students and an hour of time to fill outside of her specialism. She called them 'anorexic Tuesdays' because the dread of them was making her lose so much weight. She says she became gaunt, that she started to have suicidal feelings. 'I was a lecturer being bullied by my students,' she tells me. 'You end up praying. I got on my knees and prayed. *Please just let me die.*'

She was delivering a seminar when the Head of School knocked on the classroom door. 'You need to come to HR with me. Right now.'

The issue, they explained, was that Molly hadn't declared on her application that she had a mental illness. She also hadn't declared that she'd been sacked from a job. And yet here it was in black and white – included in her article was Molly's account of her time working as a medical receptionist, her belief that someone put spy equipment in the fax machine, and all of the subsequent fallout. Molly was asked if she had anything to say for herself. She did. She said that she used to take medication but then realised there was no such thing as schizophrenia and so stopped. She said she didn't have a mental illness. Then: 'Actually, I have superpowers. I'm like a shaman.'

Her manager explained that they didn't think she was coping with the scandal that had been created on Facebook and that they had a duty of care not to put her under that pressure.

As she cleared her desk, her colleagues kept their heads down. She was walked off the premises, devastated.

The thickness, the bitterness

Molly laughs and shakes her head. 'My next flat was so small you could be having a shit and cooking your pasta at the same time.'

Refusing to be defeated, she continued her search for work. It's how she ended up living in a rundown neighbourhood of inner-city Birmingham, doing PR for a band and grappling with an article for *Vice* magazine. By now her thoughts were starting to seriously unravel again. The familiar fears that she was a criminal – a fugitive on the run – were returning. In a moment of clarity, Molly tried to arrange to see a GP. She had been off antipsychotic medication for several months, but spurred on by a rare visit from her dad she thought perhaps she'd try taking it again. She went to a local doctors' surgery to register but it was so overrun and busy that she never made an appointment.

That's when the *Daily Mirror* launched its hate campaign. She was Britain's most wanted criminal. Vigilante groups were out to get revenge. The books in her local bookshop were all about her and her sick, dysfunctional family.

She was a danger to others, and terrified for herself.

There was only one option left. Keeping her head down so that she wouldn't be recognised, Molly took the short walk from her flat to the supermarket. 'I thought I'd drink bleach because once it was in me I wouldn't be able to get it out,' she explains.

For the first time in our conversations Molly becomes tearful. It's painful for her to talk about, and it's painful to hear.

If one good thing came out of that evening, it was that a single glimmer of light found its way into the blackness of Molly's thoughts.

She didn't see it until after she had swallowed down half a mug of bleach, vomited, drunk the rest, and sat down on her bed waiting to die. But in the minutes that followed, it occurred to Molly that there are people in this world who would help someone even if they were a hated criminal. She was only twenty-nine years old. People did reform, they did rehabilitate. Maybe – for all the terrible things she had done – there was still hope for her.

She got up, walked to the communal phone in the hallway and, with her throat now burning, dialled 999.

In A & E, Molly was X-rayed to check that she wasn't pregnant (as drinking the bleach could have harmed an unborn baby). She was put on an analgesic drip to soothe the pain. She was given milk to drink. She was fortunate that no permanent damage had been caused.

After twelve hours or so, at six o'clock in the morning, she wanted a cigarette. She was too afraid to talk to anyone and decided to step outside to see if there were any butts on the ground.

She stood at the door, taking deep breaths, psyching herself up for the media circus that she knew would be outside with their cameras and microphones, waiting to catch a glimpse of her – the captured criminal. She stepped out into the silence of the early morning. She looked around. It made no sense.

When Molly was physically well enough to leave A & E, she was placed in a wheelchair with a blanket across her knees and wheeled up the ramp into a transport ambulance.

She had no idea where she was being taken.

They drove across town, arriving at an old red-brick building. She was taken inside. Her first impression was that the corridor smelled of piss. Her first encounter was with an elderly woman whose teeth were rotting. The woman asked Molly what she was doing there. Molly told her that she was Britain's Most Wanted and the woman howled with laughter.

Molly spent a week in the psychiatric hospital.

She frequently phoned her dad, begging him to come and take her home, telling him that it felt like a prison, that she couldn't stand it.

When she was discharged, having been re-established on a medication regime, she went to stay for a bit with her dad and his girlfriend. Nurses from a community mental health team came to visit Molly and she pressed them to hand over her medical notes. She needed to piece together what had been going on. She also wanted confirmation of her diagnosis. The 'mild' had now been dropped. She was told it was 'paranoid schizophrenia'.

It was a crushing blow. Molly felt that it was the end of her life. She would never get a boyfriend again, never work again. Her dad talked about building a self-contained extension to his house where Molly could live on benefits and they could keep an eye on her.

This was it. Life was over.

If bizarre and persecutory thoughts have been a prevailing feature of Molly's mindset, equally so is her resolve.

Molly stayed at her dad's for about a month, then got back on with it. In the seven years since, she has continued to work successfully as a freelance writer and editor.

Today, as we eat pizza together in her kitchen, Molly shows me an article that she wrote five years ago for the *Daily Mail*. It's about online dating for people with mental health problems. There is a large photograph of her and the headline: 'Single female writer. 31. GSOH, schizophrenic. WLTM similar'.

It was shortly after she wrote it that she met her partner. They were both volunteering for a charity offering support for people with criminal convictions who are facing stigma.

Molly has never fully shaken the thought that she might have committed crimes; it's always there at the back of her mind. But she has reconciled herself to this. And at the same time she believes that she does have psychosis. I suggest that it must be strange to hold both of those thoughts at once.

She shrugs. 'Yeah. It is. But I'm not disturbed by it.'

And so I leave Molly, undisturbed, to press on with her day.

Driving home, my thoughts circle around that final moment of our conversation. What does it mean for a person to understand that their beliefs are detached from reality, and how might this self-knowledge interact with and shape those beliefs?

Such questions sit right at the heart of how we understand psychosis.

Let's think about that now.

Insight

ONE HUNDRED AND FIFTY years ago a twenty-year-old woman named Ann Dines was admitted to Bethlem Royal Hospital (aka 'Bedlam') in South London for psychiatric treatment. According to her medical notes she was suffering from 'insanity due to disappointment in love'.

There's a small ripple of laughter across the lecture theatre as Anthony David, Professor of Cognitive Neuropsychiatry at King's College London, shares this part of his anecdote.[1] I imagine such a diagnosis probably sounds a bit silly to some of the assembled crowd, many of whom are psychiatric professionals and researchers – though in my opinion it's actually a pretty good diagnosis, containing, as it does, at least an attempt to identify a *cause*. Not much in life has the power to hurt or consume us so much as disappointment in love.

The mood in the lecture hall seems suddenly to change as Professor David shows the next slide in his presentation. It contains a striking black-and-white photograph of Ann Dines during her time in hospital. She's slight of frame, with a thick shawl wrapped across her shoulders. Her cheeks are a little sunken, her eyes are dark and almost painfully intense. She's no longer simply a case study, not a curious artefact from the past or an amusing-sounding diagnosis. In a split second she's become a real person. And she is suffering. On her head sits a crown, fashioned from twigs and sticks. Her 'insanity' was to believe she was the Queen.

The image was taken by Hugh W. Diamond (1809–86), a physician and keen photographer who hypothesised that the cutting-edge technology of photography might be helpful in the treatment of his psychiatric patients. His idea was to show them portraits of themselves when unwell and so guide them towards 'an accurate self-image'. To encourage Ann Dines to grant her permission to be photographed Dr Diamond explained that it was his wish to take portraits of all the queens under his care, at which she immediately scoffed with contempt: 'Queens indeed! How did they obtain their titles?'

Dr Diamond conceded that they imagined them, but added that this was also the case for herself.

'No!' she said sharply. 'I never imagine such foolish delusions, they are to be pitied, but *I* was born a Queen.'[2]

Here's a fancy word: *anosognosia*. It means having as a symptom of a disorder the belief that you do not have the disorder. It's sometimes seen in people who have suffered a stroke or other neurological trauma. In so-called schizophrenia an ostensibly similar phenomenon (in its presentation, if not its cause) is generally referred to as 'lack of insight' and is entangled with the experience of delusions.

A curious truth illustrated all those years ago with Ann Dines, and played out countless times since, is that it's perfectly possible for a person locked within a delusional state to witness other people who are experiencing identical delusions and to conclude that *they* are confused, mistaken or unwell – and yet not be able to take the final logical step to infer that this must also be the case for themselves. But let's be careful not to compartmentalise this. What I'm talking about here is not some unique deficit suffered only by those of us with 'mental illness'. Insight (or a lack thereof) is part of *all* of our conscious lives *all* of the time. When comparing ourselves to others it's a fairly universal human trait that we single ourselves out for special treatment.* Let's take the example offered by Anthony David of a research study exploring the attitudes of doctors towards receiving gifts and other promotions from pharmaceutical companies. The study found that 61 per cent of the participating doctors believed that their own prescribing habits were not personally affected by such things, whereas only 16 per cent believed that their colleagues would be similarly unaffected.[3] (The laughter that evoked in the lecture theatre felt a little more cautious.)

In 1952 the Russian psychoanalyst Gregory Zilboorg wrote: 'Amongst the unclarities which are of utmost clinical importance and which cause utmost confusion is the term insight.'[4] It's an observation that still resonates today. Defining insight in the context of 'mental illness' is far from straightforward. For a start, different professional disciplines often think about it very differently.

If you were to enter the counselling room of a private psychotherapist (soft furnishings, framed artwork, a couple of rugs in earthy tones, and from somewhere the faint smell of incense) you might come to understand insight as a sort of evolving emotional and intellectual awareness of how events from your past are influencing your current thoughts, emotions and behaviours.

If, on the other hand, you were to find yourself in the consulting room of an inner-city NHS acute psychiatric ward (strip lights, plastic chairs, a potted plant with sickly looking leaves, and from

---

* As wonderfully evidenced in 'illusory superiority', a seemingly universal condition of cognitive bias whereby people (who would not be considered 'delusional' or 'mentally ill') tend to overestimate their own qualities and abilities, in relation to the same qualities and abilities of other people. This is sometimes called 'The Lake Wobegon effect' after the fictional town created by Garrison Keillor where 'all the women are strong, all the men are good-looking, and all the children are above average'.

somewhere the faint smell of cannabis) then the concept of insight might very well be reduced to how much you agree with the staff that you're 'unwell' and will be compliant with treatment. If you agree, that's good insight. If you don't, that's poor insight. It's a problematic stance, not least because of the profoundly subjective nature of psychiatry. In a candid interview with me, the psychiatrist and world-leading expert in schizophrenia research Professor Robin M. Murray offered a revealing anecdote from his own career. It concerned a psychotic patient who had been in and out of hospital many times and received several different diagnoses. A junior doctor had explained the history to Professor Murray: 'He's been in hospital four times diagnosed with schizophrenia, and three times with bipolar, and twice as schizoaffective.' Professor Murray replied, 'Oh this is ridiculous. It's as clear as a bell that this is bipolar disorder. Who on earth are these psychiatrists who thought the patient had schizophrenia?' At this point the junior doctor's lips began to quiver. 'Well, Professor,' he explained, 'I'm afraid you were one of them.'[5]

The question of precisely how psychiatric diagnoses are arrived at will be discussed later in this book. For now, my point is simply that with so much open to interpretation it's arguably a bit of a stretch – even unkind – to frame disagreement on the part of the most deeply invested person in the room as evidence of some pathological notion of 'impaired insight'.

Professor Aubrey Lewis, widely credited with raising the worldwide profile of psychiatry after the Second World War, defined insight as 'a correct attitude to morbid change in oneself' but also had the, well, insight to add that the terms 'correct', 'attitude', 'morbid' and 'change' each demand further discussion, and highlighted 'the unavoidable subjective bias in interpretations'.[6] Moreover, such broad-brush approaches ignore important subtleties. As we learnt from the experience of Molly in the previous chapter, insight is by no means binary. It doesn't have an on/off switch. It's possible for a person to have a general awareness and belief that they are 'mentally unwell', and indeed be able to name and speak at length about their delusional symptoms, while still on some level believing in the veracity of them. Investigating this multi-dimensional aspect to insight, with its plurality of concurrent awarenesses, may prove crucial to truly understanding it.

R. D. Laing described schizophrenia as 'a special strategy that a person invents in order to live in an unlivable situation'.[7] Maybe Ann Dines with her crown of twigs and sticks needed to be queen for a while, huh? To be important, to compensate for a broken heart and unbearable feelings of inadequacy. We might then frame 'poor insight' as inexorably linked to this. It wouldn't do to be crazy on top of everything else. Not like those other poor patients. The ones who *imagined* their royal titles.

It's also possible – as revealed in one of Professor Anthony David's experiments using functional Magnetic Resonance Imaging (fMRI) – that a lack of insight in people diagnosed with schizophrenia may be rooted in subtle deficits of function within cortical midline structures of the brain (which we know play a crucial role in the whole curious business of human self-awareness).[8] However, as with most studies in neuroscience, only a very small number of participants were tested; an issue that's been proven to seriously undermine the reliability of research across the field.[9] I stress this because I'm aware there's something seductive about the idea that the phenomenon we call mental illness can be explained away as biological aberrations or chemical imbalances in the brain. We, the public, do gravitate towards such explanations and may be disproportionately inclined to put our faith in them – especially, it turns out, when they're accompanied by technical-looking images.

In an experiment conducted at Colorado State University, undergraduates were asked to read genuine neuroscience papers and also a series of fake papers that made unsubstantiated claims such as 'watching television increases maths skills'. The students' ratings of their agreement with the various conclusions showed that they were consistently more likely to believe findings that were presented alongside a coloured image of the human brain, even when these findings were implausible.[10]

I suspect that one reason we find neuroscientific explanations so appealing is because however fiendishly complicated the actual science might be, it still seems to simplify everything: no need to worry about 'mental illness' because the really clever people are all over it. Except they're not. Not yet anyway. Strongly evidenced biological markers (that is to say, measurable biological characteristics that are indicative of a particular disease), as anticipated by scientists for decades, remain – at best – distant.[11] And that assumes they're there to be found.

That said, all of our life experiences, everything we think and feel and do, and our every social interaction is all etched onto our brain tissue somewhere. We've known this for millennia. 'From nothing else but thence come joys, delights, laughter and sports, and sorrows, griefs, despondency, and lamentations,' wrote Hippocrates in his musings on the human brain. 'And by the same organ we become mad and delirious, and fears and terrors assail us.'[12]

There's no ghost in the machine. There's nothing *more* to us than our brain. So it's a reasonable place to be looking.

We'll revisit some of the subtle brain changes that may play a part in psychosis in due course. For now, it's enough to caution that even our best technologies are brutally crude in the context of our bafflingly intricate neurocircuitry. The most powerful fMRI scanners can still only localise activity within regions measuring in the millimetres, which might sound small, but given that an area of brain that size will comprise something like one hundred thousand individual neurons doing all manner of different things it hardly constitutes an extreme close-up.[13] It's a point illustrated by the neuroscientist David Eagleman, who compares today's brain images with blurry pictures of earth taken from space. We're only seeing the colours and the really big stuff. In the future that will doubtless improve. We'll go Google Maps! We'll be able to zoom in ever closer and see unimaginable detail.[14] Follow this to its logical conclusion and the 'environmental' and 'neurobiological' theories will be beautifully reconciled. We'll be able to see the exact wiring that went awry when a person was frightened, bullied or abused. Or was disappointed in love.

In this version of the future our cumbersome catch-all terms like 'depression', 'anxiety' and 'schizophrenia' will have been long relegated to history, replaced with ever more precise (and doubtless still contentious) disorders of our microcircuitry. Then in a lecture theatre (on a space colony) an audience (dressed in shiny silver) will hear such antiquated terms and laugh at us.

As for Ann Dines, it seems that looking at the photographs of herself may have helped. Hugh W. Diamond recorded at the time: 'Her subsequent amusement in seeing the portraits and her frequent conversation about them was the first decided step in her gradual improvement . . . she was discharged perfectly cured, and laughed heartily at her former imaginations.'

So a happy ending from history.

But increased insight of this kind doesn't always result in increased happiness. And accepting a psychiatric diagnosis too often goes hand in hand with diminished hope and lower self-esteem,[15] which brings us to our next thorny topic.

Stigma and Discrimination

IT HAD MADE ME FEEL SO SAD to learn that upon seeing the word 'psychotic' in her medical notes (during what should have been a routine smear test) Molly began to question herself, to wonder if she might be a bad person, might even be capable of harming her baby if she became a mother. Not because she'd ever hurt anyone before but because she *associated* the word so strongly with acts of violence.

Then when she was eventually diagnosed with paranoid schizophrenia she believed her life to be as good as over. That she would never get a boyfriend or a job or live independently ever again.

'I'm not immune from the myths,' Molly explained to me. 'And the things I'd read in the paper, I kind of believed. It wasn't until later on, until I'd settled down on medication, started speaking to other people and reading more mental health-savvy literature that I started to think: hang on, maybe this isn't correct, maybe this isn't the truth.'[1] Even then, as she began to educate herself, Molly still had to deal with the prejudices of her family and her employers. It's an uncomfortable truth that for some people diagnosed with 'serious mental illness' the reactions of the people around them are more distressing than the condition itself.

Before we go on then, this seems a good time to make it clear that the overwhelming majority of people diagnosed with schizophrenia are not violent. On the contrary, their vulnerability puts them at a significantly greater risk of being the victims of violence. One American study revealed that people diagnosed with schizophrenia were fourteen times more likely to be the victim of a

violent crime than to be arrested for one.[2] The common perception of people with schizophrenia being a danger to society is
wholly inaccurate.

This is also a good time to stress that what we call schizophrenia
needn't be a life sentence. There are complications in pinning down
the exact rates of recovery, not least because recovery is a concept
that means different things to different people. For some, it might
mean a complete remission of 'clinical symptoms'. For others, it will
be a journey; a subjective improvement of wellbeing and growth,
and of staying in control of life. This might involve the attribution of
meaning to experiences over time, rather than returning to an earlier mindset. There are also those who reject the very concept of
mental health recovery on moral and philosophical grounds. Such
is the position of the user-led campaign group Recovery in the Bin,
who argue that the term has been co-opted by the mental health
system as a means to further discipline and control people. They
believe that autonomy and self-determination, at the heart of any
true recovery, cannot be calibrated by outcome measures.[3]

All that said, if we decide not to reject the term, then by any
metric so far proposed – be it clinical or more deeply personal –
meaningful and sustained recovery from so-called schizophrenia
can and frequently does happen.[4]

'Popular knowledge about mental illness', writes Graham Thornicroft, 'is a potent cocktail of profound ignorance and pernicious
misinformation.'[5]

I first met Graham when I was making a radio documentary
about mental health and the media. He is Professor of Community
Psychiatry at King's College London and a world-leading expert
on the subject of mental health stigma.

I'll lay my cards on the table. When I first set out to write this book, I decided that I'd try and get to the end without mentioning stigma at all.

I find it a bit troubling how the subject of stigma has come to dominate so much of our discourse on mental health, especially via social media. A lot of this is led by (granted, well-meaning) high-profile individuals and celebrities who talk and tweet and post messages about mental health *stigma* and the problem with *stigma* and the need to reduce *stigma*. And the whole time we might just be looking in the wrong direction.

It's a conclusion reached by Graham Thornicroft, too. 'The trouble with stigma', he explains, 'is that it's such a vague, fuzzy concept and it hasn't left us able to do anything to reduce social exclusion.' He reflects on a story from his own life. When he was just three years old, his mother sank into a painful depression. Graham went to live with his grandparents while she was given a series of treatments. The drugs didn't help her at all, he says, but she was eventually given electroconvulsive therapy (ECT), which did help her a great deal, and a year after his mother first became unwell the family was reunited. Graham's mother was employed as a district nurse but for the whole time that she was undergoing those treatments she never told anybody at her work about what she was going through, or why she needed time off. She was afraid that if she did she would be treated as damaged goods, that her position at work would become precarious. That was over fifty years ago, yet it's a fear many people still have today, and not without foundation. Every year in the UK three hundred thousand people lose their jobs due to mental health issues.[6]

'People's life experiences are being limited', says Graham Thornicroft, 'because of public and occupational perceptions.'

So now we have something to tease apart because what we're really talking about mightn't be stigma at all.

Stigma refers to a person's feelings of shame, disgrace or inadequacy due to their circumstances. Getting sacked from work could certainly lead to such feelings. So too could being shunned or ridiculed by those around us. But in these scenarios stigma is the *result*, not the *cause*. The psychologists Anne Cooke and Dave Harper argue that stigma individualises what may in fact be issues of prejudice and discrimination.

'We don't talk about the stigma of being a woman, or of being black,' they explain. 'We talk, quite rightly, about sexism and racism.'[7]

Why then are we so quick to internalise matters where our mental health is concerned? Well, one theory is that the current raft of public education and anti-stigma campaigns actively encourages us to think in this way.

In 2016, the BBC ran a season of programming on its flagship BBC One channel called *In the Mind*. Announcing this schedule, James Harding, Director of BBC News, said: 'This is a moment when we stop and reflect on one of the big issues of our time, one that touches all of us. We will report and examine – with all the BBC's expertise, insight and understanding – on what's really happening in mental health.'[8] There were documentaries, a mental health-related story-line on *EastEnders* and a series of other news and talk-show items. One of the most high-profile programmes in this schedule was a documentary presented by the celebrated actor, comedian and all-round national treasure Stephen Fry, entitled *The Not So Secret Life of the Manic Depressive: 10 Years On.* This was a sequel to the 2006 Emmy award-winning documentary *Stephen Fry: The Secret Life of a Manic Depressive,* in which Fry talked about his own painful difficulties in experiencing very high and low moods.

The sequel begins with footage of Stephen Fry in 2012 in Kampala, Uganda, where he was filming another documentary, interviewing the Ugandan Ethics and Integrity Minister, Simon Lokodo – who in Fry's inimitable words was 'a foaming, frothing homophobe of the worst kind'. He had proposed a bill to make homosexuality a capital offence. In the footage we see Lokodo jabbing a threatening finger towards Fry, a gay man, and shouting him down, stating that he will be arrested if he tries to promote his homosexuality or recruit others, and so on. All vile, nasty stuff. Fry is visibly shaken as he leaves the interview.

Cut to the present day and Stephen Fry is in the office of his psychiatrist, Dr William Shanahan. Together they recount the events that followed that distressing encounter. Fry recalls how he returned to his hotel feeling the lowest he had ever felt. 'I paced around trying to analyse what it was that had disappeared from me. It seemed as though the whole essence of me had disappeared. Everything that was me was no longer there. Just some feeling came over me that this was the end.'

He had vodka and also pills of some kind in his room. 'I just carefully lined up I don't know how many of those damned pills,' he says, 'and drank all the vodka that there was there with the pills. The next thing I remember was that I'm on the floor, [and] an embarrassed member of the hotel is looking down at the carpet in the doorway [saying], "We've just got to get him to a hospital."'

Back in the UK two days later, Fry decided he needed to see a psychiatrist. 'I have a dim memory of arriving here,' he says, at which point Dr Shanahan takes over: 'When you arrived, let me remind you [you were] sorry that you were still alive. And wanting to die. And feeling that you should have died.'

So a truly horrible experience for a person to suffer. And we learn that Fry was admitted for a short stay in hospital.

'At the age of fifty-six,' a narrator tells us, 'Stephen got a formal mental health diagnosis of cyclothymia, mood swings that lead to disturbed behaviour. But with the diagnosis came the medication and that immediately made him feel much better.'

End of scene.

Watching this documentary at the time, it seemed odd to me that no airtime was given over to the psychiatrist discussing the possibility with Stephen Fry that his plummeting mood and desperate cry for help were likely to be connected to the terrible thing that had just happened to him.

He had been thousands of miles from the safety and security of his home, on a presumably gruelling work schedule, and was forced to try to defend his very existence to a hideous and powerful man, who from the comfort of a ministerial office took delight in humiliating and threatening him, and – let's not fuck about here – ultimately wished him dead.

Now possibly none of that is enough to fully explain why Stephen Fry drank the vodka and took those pills, but I would argue that it almost certainly played a part.

We have no idea what private conversations were shared between doctor and patient when the cameras weren't rolling. Quite probably they did talk at length about such things. I hope so. My point is that the BBC TV programme did not.

Following its broadcast there was some criticism levied against the BBC. An open letter written to the broadcaster by Peter Kinderman, Professor of Psychology at Liverpool University, and over one thousand other signatories – including high-profile academics, mental health professionals and mental health service users – stated that although the Fry documentary and other programmes in the *In the Mind* season were clearly well intentioned, they made the mistake of taking for granted the contested view that mental health problems are necessarily a manifestation of biological illness.

The letter criticised:

. . . a failure to acknowledge that the origins of problems, and the things that keep them going, are often not simply in the brain but in the events and circumstances of people's lives – including poverty, urban living, migration, childhood abuse, bullying, racism and other forms of victimisation. This has been confirmed by a vast volume of research, and the evidence is in fact stronger than for the involvement of biological factors. Educating the public about this would not only increase understanding: research suggests that this kind of approach reduces stigma and, in many cases, is more helpful for those affected.[9]

Needless to say, fewer people have read the letter than watched the TV shows.

'Look at the politicians and policy makers shouting loudest about anti-stigma,' says psychologist and author Dr Lucy Johnstone. 'They're the very people who are reinforcing the policies that are driving people crazy.'[10]

Like many people who have made mental health their life's work, Lucy Johnstone experienced more than her fair share of distress as a child and adolescent. She's the sort of person whose way of coping with that was to lock herself away in her bedroom and voraciously read. This was the late 1970s when the anti-psychiatry movement was at full throttle. An idealist at heart, she was still in her twenties and a recently qualified clinical psychologist when she wrote her first book, *Users and Abusers of Psychiatry*. She's been writing and working in the field ever since. I meet with her in our shared hometown of Bristol, where our talk quickly turns political – because if it's impossible to speak about mental health without talking about stigma, it's equally impossible to seriously consider stigma without talking politics.

'Every single government seems to have leapt on the anti-stigma campaigns,' argues Johnstone. 'Theresa May among others. But what are they doing to stop people being targeted by the benefits office? To the huge increase in inequality? The rise of zero-hours jobs? These are the things that drive people mad. It's no kind of answer to say that as long as we're happy to say we've got a mental illness we're making progress. It's absolute nonsense. It's insulting. And it's politically motivated. Does the current government or the previous one want to talk about discrimination? No, they don't. Do they want to make themselves look very well-meaning by talking about anti-stigma? Yes, they do.'

Since 2007, the Department of Health in England has provided funding for the Time to Change initiative: a national programme to reduce mental health stigma and discrimination, led by the charities Mind and Rethink Mental Illness. I've been involved in some of their work myself over the years, including the annual Time to Talk Day – encouraging more public conversations about our mental health and wellbeing.

That's got to be helpful, right?

Yes. Obviously, I think so or else I wouldn't get involved. But I'm also concerned that the emphasis of such campaigns too often seems to begin and end with raising awareness, while doing little to improve knowledge. Sure, it's a good thing if someone feels less inhibited about disclosing to a friend or colleague that they're having difficulties. But if those difficulties are extremely serious – if they're feeling hopeless, if their life feels unlivable, if they can see no way out – then it's no easy thing for their friend or colleague to know how to respond, let alone how to get the right help.*

Even so, Time to Change almost certainly does help some people who are experiencing mental health difficulties by improving the attitudes of others. It's tax-funded so it needs to prove its worth. On its website it reports: 'Our national surveys show the overall attitude trend between 2008 and 2016 was positive with a 9.6% change – that's an estimated 4.1m people with improved attitudes.'[11] That sounds pretty good. Though I'd suggest that a single number valuation assigned to a variable as nuanced as 'improved attitudes' demands a bit of unpacking.

If we dig into some of the surveys underpinning this figure, as Professor Graham Thornicroft and colleagues have done, we will see that no distinction is made between more common mental health diagnoses and less common ones. So we should not assume, for instance, that any changes in public attitudes apply equally to something as culturally laden with damning stereotypes as 'schizophrenia' as they do to more commonly experienced and talked about mental health problems such as 'depression' or 'anxiety'.[12]

In fact, the *It's an illness like any other and you wouldn't tell me to pull myself together if I had cancer/a broken leg/diabetes* message (which forms the bedrock of almost all mental health anti-stigma campaigns) may actually *increase* prejudice against people with a schizophrenia diagnosis because although we're less inclined to blame people for their strange behaviours if we believe they're suffering from a brain disease, we're also more likely to fear and

---

* If you are concerned that someone you know might be considering ending their life by suicide and you don't know what to say or do about it, there's an excellent training resource created by the Zero Suicide Alliance. It's free to do. It takes twenty minutes. You can find it on their website: https://zerosuicidealliance.com/

avoid them and to see them as dangerous and unpredictable.[13]

It's for these reasons that many people (including, I would imagine, many of the thousand-plus signatories of the BBC complaint) reject the standard government-endorsed anti-stigma message, along with its biological and medical assumptions.

There are also plenty of reasons why the government might be rather keen to stick with it. Aligning themselves with the biomedical model of mental distress means that they're not stuck with the irksome problem of how to deal with bizarre and disturbing behaviour that doesn't fall under the remit of criminal law. More convenient, perhaps, to label it as a 'medical problem' (just like cancer and diabetes!) and so effectively remove it from governmental jurisdiction.[14]

It's a complicated situation that cannot be adequately communicated with a simple, celebrity-spearheaded soundbite.

The truth is that mental illness isn't remotely like a broken leg.

However, we should be cautious not to throw the biological baby out with the sociopolitical bath water.* The physical/mental health analogy mightn't be completely flawed.

As the psychiatrist and blogger Dr Alex Langford explains, a diabetes comparison to mental health problems is actually pretty useful so long as we focus on Type 2 diabetes. He compares this to depression:

> Whereas Type 1 always involves the same underlying problem – destruction of pancreas cells leading to a lifelong need for insulin – Type 2 is a more variable biological state, just like

---

* I always bathe my children in sociopolitical bath water. It's surprisingly gentle on the skin and makes bathtime conversations infinitely more interesting.

depression. In Type 2 diabetes, high sugar levels are primarily caused by the body not being as responsive to insulin as it should be, but insulin levels are often low as well. Other hormones like glucagon and incretin are out of kilter too. This is akin to depression, in which we know that it's not just serotonin that's important at the biological level. Other neurotransmitters like noradrenalin and dopamine (and many others) are all involved . . . Also, neither Type 2 diabetes nor depression have one simple cause. Both are caused by a collection of individually small risk factors. With diabetes the big dangers are things like obesity, high cholesterol, poor diet and sedentary lifestyle, whereas with depression it's things like recent adverse life events, a tough childhood and a lack of social support. Diabetes and depression both have a huge genetic component, but neither has a single-gene cause.

So there are certainly some similarities.

Also, by considering depression and diabetes in this way Langford notes the irony of some people still insisting that those of us with mental health issues should *pull ourselves together*. He comments, 'It's probably easier to shift your Type 2 diabetes by avoiding junk food, exercising and losing weight than it is to ease your depression by taking away life stressors like a busy job and magically undoing an abusive childhood.'[15]

But what to do about mental health stigma?

Well, Dr Lucy Johnstone has a pretty radical suggestion: 'The quickest and easiest way of getting rid of stigma is to get rid of psychiatric diagnoses.'

So we should probably talk about diagnosis.

First, let's meet a soldier.

THE SOLDIER

YOU REALISE THAT NONE of it's really true.

You were led to believe that you were someone who had great importance to the world. And then you see it was a trick. Your brain played a horrible trick on you. You feel cheated.

Then comes a yearning to find meaning. Why did I experience this? What was its purpose? How did I end up locked in a seclusion cell, howling and wailing like a caged animal? More animal than human, Mum said. Why did the army select me for this mission?

Enterprise Medical Log, Stardate 5027.3, Dr Leonard McCoy recording: I'm concerned about Captain Kirk. He shows indications of increasing tension and emotional stress. I can find no reason for the Captain's behaviour, except possibly that we've been on patrol too long without relief and diversion. He has resisted all of my attempts to run a psychological profile on him.

'I think you're unwell, Dad. It's like—' James Wooldridge sniffed hard and wiped away a rogue tear with the sleeve of his jumper. 'It's like that *Star Trek* episode when Kirk was really stressed and making the wrong decisions. He had to step down for a bit. It's like that.'

The atmosphere in the house during the past few months had been unbearably tense. James's elder brother and sister had already moved out so it was just James and his younger brother who were witnessing first-hand their parents' marriage falling apart. James suspected this was at least partly his own fault. It couldn't have helped that he so frequently woke his parents up in the middle of the night with all of his worrying. What was he even worrying about? Nuclear war. The stuff in his Gideons Bible. The way that he smelled. At school he wore a thick woollen trench coat – not dissimilar to the kind his grandad would have worn in the army – and he would push his face into the rough fabric and inhale deeply. He smelled of stale wee, he was sure of it. That kept him awake, too. But mostly it was the stuff in his Bible. *I am the way. I am the light.* Too much reading; too little sleeping. He could never seem to sleep. And waking his parents up all the time. That couldn't have helped.

So now it was down to James, at fifteen years of age, to stop his dad from abandoning them. He had to persuade him for the sake of his mum and brother. And also – mostly – for himself. He idolised his dad. Worshipped him. This man who had served as a chief technician in the RAF and who had a natural, almost breezy intelligence that James had inherited. James stood tall, fixed his dad's gaze. 'This isn't who you are,' he insisted. Or words to that effect. It's hard to remember every detail. This was over thirty-five years ago. The only memory that won't fade is his dad's response. He laughed. That's what he did. He laughed in James's face. 'You're too young to understand, son.' It was humiliating. His dad wasn't unwell. He was having an affair. His parting gift to his son was to encourage him to apply to take his A levels at Welbeck College – a specialist and highly selective institution for excellent students who intend to take up careers in the military.

'I don't blame the army,' James will tell me more than once. 'I've never blamed the army for what happened to me. If there was an inherent weakness in me, it was right that they found it.'

We've met at James's home, a cramped and cosy little cottage overlooking a picturesque church in the ancient market town of South Molton, North Devon. He welcomed me with a wry apology that if I was expecting the smell of fresh bread, I was about to be disappointed. 'We're both smokers and we've got a dog. I'll put the kettle on.' He has an air of the military about him (at least to my civilian sensibilities). He's shaved, has neatly cropped grey hair. He's also broad-shouldered, stands up straight and speaks in measured, confident tones. It's markedly different to how he sounded when we first talked on the phone a couple of months back. He was recovering from a recent relapse and had been knocked hard. He felt betrayed by himself. There was a weariness in his voice then, a resignation: 'I'm fifty-one years old. How can I still keep getting these feelings when it's becoming less and less likely that they're going to be based on truth?'

And yet as his story unfolds, I find myself struck by the truths and logic and emotional needs that seem to provide a scaffolding for his more bizarre beliefs. Beliefs that stretch back to a freezing parade square at the Royal Military Academy Sandhurst, and a desperate need to not be abandoned again.

Dorm truths

The Welbeck College Selection Board involved three days of intense scrutiny at an army barracks in Westbury. There were maths and physics exams as well as physical endurance tests, assault courses – the squeak of dozens of pairs of Dunlop Green Flash trainers on the wooden floors of old, draughty gym halls. And always they were being observed. That's what James remembers most keenly. The feeling of being observed, scrutinised, assessed.

'You were being observed even when you didn't know you were being observed,' he tells me. He remembers that one lunchtime his tie sloshed into his bowl of soup. *Shit. I bet they've seen that.* I've a sense he was observing himself more critically than even they were.

From thousands of applicants from across the Commonwealth only seventy-five students were admitted to any given cohort. 'They were looking for leadership potential,' James explains. 'Leadership potential in fifteen-year-olds.' In the final interview he stood before three uniformed men, with more watching from the sides of the room. The three men were sitting behind a long table, shuffling through his application papers. 'Your father was in the RAF, wasn't he? Why do you want to join the army?'

James's mind flickered to his dad and to everything going on at home. 'I want to keep my feet on the ground, sir.'

The officer raised an eyebrow, gave an almost imperceptible nod.

When the letter arrived, James secretly hoped for a rejection. The past few months had been unrelentingly grim. His mum had found out about his dad's affair and the environment at home had become so toxic that James had gone to live with his sister while his parents proceeded with a divorce.

He couldn't concentrate at school, lost his motivation, did less well in his O levels than everyone expected. He was feeling disconnected from life, apathetic about his future. 'I didn't care if I didn't work,' he tells me. 'I could just spend my life on the dole. I was really out of it.'

But clearly Welbeck had seen something in him that they wanted, and again it was his dad who encouraged James to accept the offer.

What James didn't know at the time was that his dad was already planning a new life for himself and his girlfriend in Saudi Arabia.

He wonders now if sending him off to a boarding college was his dad's attempt to ensure he'd be looked after in some way. 'But I don't know,' he concludes, waving the thought away. 'I don't know what he was thinking.'

On the train, James folded and unfolded a newspaper. He felt too nervous to read it, had really only bought it for show. He decided that a lot of this was going to be about appearance and it would give a sophisticated impression to arrive with a serious broadsheet tucked under his arm.

He was still to break out the other side of puberty. He was small, pigeon-chested and with a shock of curly hair that would soon earn him the nickname of Pube Head. He carried a suitcase with shiny brass buckles and wore a pinstripe three-piece suit that bunched up around his shoulders. He was still wrestling with whether he'd made the right decision, not least as it involved moving so far away from his girlfriend.

James had met Louise at school and after plucking up the courage to make her a Valentine's Day card – complete with schmaltzy poem – hadn't quite believed his luck when she'd said 'yes'. 'She was one of the best-looking girls in school,' he tells me. 'She was a quarter Italian, had a Roman nose, dark skin.' Bottom line is he really fancied her. They started dating, going to local discos, and soon things got serious. 'I was besotted, fell head over heels in love. All intense, sixteen-year-old stuff. My parents were divorcing. I think I was channelling a lot of my feelings into this relationship.'

The train arrived at Worksop station in North Nottinghamshire, from where James and a cluster of other new cadets were to take a minibus on the final leg of the journey to Welbeck Abbey, where the college was based. James kept his head down, doesn't remember sharing a single word with the other boys. But as the bus tyres crunched up the gravel driveway of the estate, he caught his first glimpse of the abbey. Even remembering this today seems to have a physical effect on him. He takes a deep breath, lets it out slowly. 'I was just in awe,' he says at last. 'It was a beautiful, *beautiful* place.'

It's a feeling that has never left him. Until then James had attended a regular comprehensive school; this was like nothing he had ever known. 'Just being with all these other intelligent, fit, bright, keen, motivated people was a real breath of fresh air from where I'd been before,' he recalls.

In talking about his English master, James draws parallels with the teacher played by Robin Williams in *Dead Poets Society*. He recalls his class being taking to a sunken garden in the grounds, where they sat beside a crescent swimming pool and the master read them poetry.

It's not remotely how I imagined a military sixth form to be. But this was intended to prepare boys to become high-ranking army officers. As well as studying for A levels there were lessons in diplomacy, letter writing, the polite times to arrive for a cocktail party, a dinner party, a breakfast meeting. When it was acceptable to be late, and how soon to be late.

The boys wore blazers and starched trousers and polished shoes, or military fatigues for assault training and parade drills. They slept in dorms, and it was here that the Dorm Truths took place. 'They were pretty cruel, in a way,' James tells me. 'Or they could be cruel. We'd go around the dorm and say the truth about every other cadet. Tell them what we really thought of them. Some lads got ripped apart if they weren't well liked.'

And what did his peers make of him?

He doesn't miss a beat: 'That I was too sensitive. And I was. I was too sensitive.' He was also self-conscious and prone to turning red if a teacher singled him out to speak in front of the class. He still felt unsettled by his parents' divorce. Over the three terms of his first year, he went home to four different houses. Then came the letter from Louise. 'My heart plummeted through the floor,' James tells me. 'I went to bed early for three or four nights in a row, just got my head under the covers and wept through the night. I suppose I was dealing with a bit of loss.'

The other lads might have called James out on his sensitivity but he was still liked and respected. After Louise dumped him a whole group of his friends offered to write to her, to try to persuade her to take him back. He didn't take them up on the offer, but he felt touched that they cared enough to suggest it. In Welbeck College, and in the promise of joining the army upon graduation, he'd found a family he could depend on.

'It felt like home,' he tells me. 'This is where I belonged now.'

Rowallan Company

James swore his allegiance to Her Majesty the Queen and signed the Official Secrets Act. At eighteen years of age, having graduated from Welbeck, he was now officially a private in the British Army. Moreover, he was an officer cadet at the Royal Military Academy Sandhurst; if he made it through to the other side he would be a second lieutenant.

This was the mid-eighties and at that time there were two routes through Sandhurst: the Standard Military Course (SMC) and the now disbanded Rowallan Company. 'Everyone knew about Rowallan,' James tells me. 'There were scare stories.' The purpose of Rowallan Company was to train up recruits who were deemed by the Army Officer Selection Board to have potential but to be 'Not Yet Ready' to take the Standard Military Course. It was essentially a twelve-week pre-selection programme.

From its official literature at the time:

> The Rowallan course has a simple objective – to develop leadership qualities. Those who pass will go on immediately to join the Standard Military Course ... The training methods originated by Lord Rowallan, consistently re-evaluated and enhanced, have produced a course that is somewhat unusual in military terms. It is designed to help the young man realise his own potential. At the end of the course, his self-confidence, self-knowledge, resilience, determination, initiative, resourcefulness and adaptability are all so developed that he has a head start when he joins the SMC ... The Rowallan course is physically and mentally demanding and some students do have difficulty in meeting the required standards. But the sense of achievement, the evident development of character and the remarkable esprit and comradeship of the company ensure that all look back on the course with gratitude and a sense of privilege.

Visit an online British Army forum and a typical recollection from a soldier who trained with Rowallan Company looks something like this: 'At the time it was utter, utter, physical and mental (particularly mental) ******* purgatory, made worse by being very young.' And another reflection of a SMC officer cadet looking in from the outside: 'No matter how bad my day was going, looking out of my window of Old/New College, seeing those guys in their natty Red Tracksuits being ragged to **** made me realise that life could be far far far worse.'

James resigned himself to the Rowallan scheme. He recalls part of his Selection Board process involved debating solutions for drug problems in society. He spoke quietly, proposed an argument that prevention was better than cure, but was shouted down by more confident public school boys and university graduates, and his contribution was lost.

He wasn't unduly concerned. In fact, he was beginning to feel a surge in his confidence. It was yet to reach the surface but he could feel it stirring in his belly. He walked in the direction of the Rowallan Company barracks, hauling his army-issue bergen. There was snow on the ground. His freshly shaved head felt cold in the freezing wind.

He looked across to the Grand Steps leading into the Old College. The steps where the adjutant marches his horse to signal the end of each Sovereign's Parade, a ceremony celebrating the passing out from Sandhurst of officer cadets, who on the stroke of midnight become commissioned officers. It's also during the Sovereign's Parade that the best, most exemplary cadet is awarded the Sword of Honour.

James could see it. He could picture it as though he were already there. He stands proudly to attention wearing his ceremonial navy blue uniform, white gloves, peaked cap. His mum and dad are looking on from the stands. No arguing today. They take hold of each other's hands for this one perfect moment as their son – singled out, special, important – salutes Her Majesty the Queen and humbly accepts the Sword of Honour.

James isn't simply going to make it through Sandhurst. He's going to be the best.

Then it starts.

The alarms sound at 0530hrs. Some of the lads sleep underneath their beds in sleeping bags rather than crease the bedsheets that must now be pulled into precision right angles for the first inspection of the day.

Fuck up and be punished.

It won't stop. It's relentless. From the moment they wake to the moment they collapse, exhausted, into sleep.

James is up already. He's washed. His bedsheets are perfect. His clothes are immaculately folded and stored in the 'tin' beside his bed. Even his socks are rolled and folded into regulation squares.

His bergen is packed and ready for whatever they throw at him. It can happen at any time: *Get your shit together and be on the truck in five minutes.* Then rattling around in the back of a four-tonne lorry to God only knows where. He needs to be ready. He is ready.

Morning drill. He's first out on the frozen parade square. He can see his breath in the gloomy darkness. He needs to be first so he can be the right marker – the soldier in the front right-hand position of the parade. Everyone will take their lead from him. It doesn't stop. There's no downtime. Breakfast is eaten as fast as possible, as much as possible. It's about fuel. Platefuls upon platefuls. Loading up with calories. Get into the canteen first; eat for the longest. Always first. Change into combats and out onto the Barossa – an expanse of bitterly cold heathlands – for endurance exercises. The straps of his bag tear into his shoulders. He's looking for paint pots – *paint pots!* – in the middle of nowhere. *Don't find them and you're sleeping outside tonight.* It's fucking with James's head. It's designed to fuck with their heads. Parallel paths, invisible from each other. Check the map again. In the map reading exam he scored higher than anyone. The grades were displayed on the wall of the barracks for all to see. He's doing this. He's the best. It doesn't stop. It's relentless. Double-march back to the barracks: lungs burning, eyes streaming. Need to be the first.

Need to be the best. The days and weeks are collapsing into each other. It doesn't stop. There's no downtime. The mundane is taking on a new dimension. Something strange and wonderful is happening. James is cleaning the brass piping of a urinal. His knees ache on the hard tile floor. He's scrubbing at the piping with a stiff toothbrush, a tin of Brasso. An instructor arrives. The instructor demonstrates the correct use of commercial cleaning products. He sinks his fingers into a tin of black boot polish. The polish is all over his fingers. He picks up a spray can, sprays it onto his hands, wipes it with a cloth. He's clean. *An army secret, a new technology.* James blinks; his eyes are stinging with tears. He looks around at his fellow cadets, grinning wildly. Did they see that? Is he the only one who gets it? He wants to laugh and shout and cry: *You bastards! Why did you never show us this before?* The days and weeks are collapsing into each other. There is a chapel in the grounds and James is in the chapel, sitting in the pews. Cold light diffuses through the stained-glass windows and a couple of rows in front are two of his peers from Welbeck College and they are singing 'Onward, Christian Soldiers' and it is the most beautiful thing James has ever heard and he is choking back tears and tears are streaming down his face and he feels the breath of God. He is in a lecture theatre and the days and weeks are collapsing into each other and James is standing at the front of the lecture theatre and he is talking and talking and talking and how this happened was that the officer was lecturing them on how to be officers and James put his hand up and asked, *How do you expect us to develop as officers when each of us is training to be an officer and so everybody wants to be the person in charge?* and the officer said, *Good point, why don't you tell us what your thoughts are?* and maybe James was supposed to speak from his seat but what he did – what he found himself doing –

was walking to the front and he didn't stand behind the lectern because it's important not to put a barrier between yourself and your audience and he told them that but now he has lost his thread and he no longer knows what he's talking about and he is talking about his knee because before Sandhurst he injured his knee and it was an old rugby injury and the other cadets are fidgeting in their seats and looking at each other and James is explaining how his knee is giving him problems when he feels the firm clasp of the officer's hand on his shoulder and the officer is saying, *Perhaps we ought to give your knee a rest now.* – Yes, sir! The days and weeks are collapsing into each other. It's late and Rowallan Company are in the dormitory polishing their boots and mopping the floors and there's a cadet sitting on his bed listening to his Walkman and everyone hates that guy because he never pulls his weight and *look at him nodding his head like a fucking idiot and not pulling his weight again* and James is reaching into his kit bag and pulling out his machete and he's walking across the dorm towards the cadet who is listening to his Walkman and hasn't noticed that the dormitory has fallen silent.

James pulls the machete from its sheath and in one gesture holds the blade to the face of the cadet, an inch from his chin.

They stare at each other.

It doesn't stop. There's no downtime. It's night and James lies awake on his bed and listens to the snores and grunts and farts of the other cadets but he won't sleep because he will be ready for anything and he will be awarded the Sword of Honour. The alarms sound at 0530hrs for a parade drill but James has packed away the uniform that his parade sergeant is telling them they need to wear. It's deep in the bottom of his bergen. He packed it to be ready. But now he isn't ready and the other cadets are getting dressed before him. He ties his laces, pulls on his beret. He pushes past them. He needs to be first to be the right marker. He stands to attention on the freezing parade square. He's the first. It's still dark. He watches his breath escape in clouds. He feels dizzy, euphoric. The sergeant is telling him to leave the parade and as he marches back towards the barracks he holds his head high.

Everyone is watching. They can all see how special and important he is, as he marches across the parade square, still wearing his pyjamas.

He's lasted five weeks.

Psychological weaponry

He had to think straight. This was part of a test and he needed to plan his escape. That made sense. Just as it made sense that the grounds of Sandhurst were unusually empty of life this morning, as James, dressed in his civilian clothes, was escorted by a corporal to return his uniform, and to sign some paperwork in the commanding officer's office with its grey metal filing cabinets.

He had no idea he was signing his own discharge papers. He was signing things all the time at Sandhurst. That was nothing unusual. Besides, he had no reason to think he was being kicked out.

He was the best cadet by a stretch.

The corridors and parade squares were deserted because his top-secret mission was soon to start and the other soldiers couldn't be party to what was happening.

And now he was in the guard room, staring at maps on the walls. The control panels were filled with dials and buttons and security monitors. He needed to think straight and to control his breathing.

He couldn't control his breathing. Why was it so hard to breathe? His eyes stung with tears, he couldn't get enough air in his lungs.

He was hyperventilating. He tore at his shirt.

The door opened hard, slamming against the wall. The big bastard provo sergeant stormed in, gripped a hand round James's throat, pinned him against the wall. 'What the fuck is wrong with you?' he demanded.

'Nothing. Nothing. Nothing,' James replied.

James was detained in the guard room at Sandhurst for eight hours. During this time he was given nothing to eat or drink.

For a while he was placed in an adjoining dormitory and told to rest, but his head was all over the place, and in any case he felt too hungry to sleep. Different people came and went. He recalls that for a while he shared the dorm with a group of Gurkhas. 'Four or five of them came in,' he tells me. 'They were speaking in Gorkhali. I was trying to match them. In my own mind I was conversing with them.'

James doesn't speak Gorkhali. Looking back, he feels they understood he was unwell. He felt a deep and genuine empathy from these men and was calmer in their presence.

His memories after that are patchy at best. At some point he was told that his mum had arrived. He was escorted outside to her car. She was there with his elder brother. They had been given his belongings. Opening the car door, he recalls, there was a strong smell of beef and mustard sandwiches. He began ripping through bags to find them, searching out the food. He was in strict survival mode, incapable of communicating.

Later his mum would describe him as seeming more animal than human. His face looked hollow and sunken. There was a deadness behind his eyes.

James doesn't remember what words he shared with his mum and brother on that drive home. What he does remember is that the radio was on. It was BBC Radio 4, some kind of debate. 'I became part of the programme,' he explains. 'My mind took me into the role of the person that was speaking. So it was me doing the speaking. And initially this person wasn't doing very well, they were being shouted down, making mistakes, and I was battling to get it right. I was still doing my public speaking training, really trying hard to win over this audience. And then after a period some music came on. It was classical music. But once again, I was the one who was composing, conducting, playing. It was a blessed relief because I could lose myself in the music for a moment and that was like my reward for having done well in the public speaking.'

All the while James was looking out the window at the cars coming the other way. He was reading the registration plates. That one was his staff sergeant; that one the commanding officer; those were his fellow officer cadets. They were keeping tabs on him, making sure he was doing everything right.

The next day, James was taken to a hospital deep within enemy territory. He should never have let it get this far.

In the ambulance he'd let himself become confused. He believed he was being taken to a celebration. His whole family was going to be there. His dad had come home from Saudi Arabia. Louise would be there, too, and the officers and his fellow cadets from Welbeck and Sandhurst.

He'd done so well that he wouldn't need to complete his training. He was to be instantly commissioned.

Except when the ambulance arrived at North Devon District Hospital, there was nobody waiting for him. This wasn't right. Something wasn't right. For the first time, he felt frightened. He quickly gave the ambulance crew the slip, running as fast as he could, weaving across the car park and into one of the hospital buildings, along corridors, crashing through sets of double doors, up and down stairwells. He was being chased by security guards and half a dozen psychiatric nurses. They cornered him outside the morgue.

For a brief moment reality shifted and James was inside an arcade game. There was a big red button beside the locked doors to the morgue. This was the Smart Bomb; blow up everything on the screen and be transported to somewhere else.

He reached to press it, felt the first hands grab hold of him.

He was dragged onto a ward, restrained on a bed. There were people holding his arms and legs, someone else holding his head. He couldn't move. He was terrified. He felt the needle go in.

For the first few days and weeks, James battled to stay awake. He needed to remain alert and be aware of his environment. This was an unsafe place. He couldn't risk sleeping. But the medication they were giving him – a thick orange syrup in small plastic cups – made him more tired than he'd ever felt in his life. He had no energy to lift his legs. He shuffled along the corridor to the patient kitchen, where he pressed a trembling hand onto the metal surfaces to help keep his balance. He ate instant coffee by the spoonful.

He was dribbling. His hands shook to the point that he couldn't hold a knife and fork. When he went to the toilet his guts were like water or else he was so constipated it was all he could do to not cry out with the pain.

He needed to work out what was happening. He had his theories. Most likely the army was testing a new kind of psychological weaponry and had selected him as a strong, top cadet to road-test it.

He must have been given something at Sandhurst to make him go mad, and now he had to overcome it – return from the brink – and infiltrate psychiatric services. As a soldier in the guise of a patient he was tasked to ensure that this place was fit and proper for service personnel.

James's incarceration lasted several months. In his worse moments he wasn't sure if he was alive or what, if anything, was real.

Placing his hands under cold water felt real. Ten, maybe twenty times a day he would hide away from the staff and stand at his bedroom sink with his hands under the taps, washing away a bad energy. He filled a jug with his urine and drank it. He dug his fingernails into his palms until the skin ripped open; he punched and kicked at the walls and the doors, howling and screaming.

Some of these tests were to prove he was alive. Others were intended to push his body to its limits, a continuation of his military training.

'To a certain extent you relive it as you retell it,' James told me the first time we spoke, when he was still feeling bruised and wary from his most recent relapse. 'There are some experiences from when I've been unwell that I'm still coming to terms with.'

As we talk today we move back and forth through his life. He's been admitted to hospital multiple times. He recalls that during that first admission, when he was still just a teenager, his mum visited him every day. She brought him in bottles of milk – his favourite drink – and would sit and worry with him for hours at a time.

He told her to fuck off. It wasn't *her* he wanted.

He still regrets that. Hates how much it must have hurt her. 'I do love my mum dearly, don't get me wrong. But at the time—'

'You wanted your dad?' I venture.

'I wanted my dad. I really did. I was crying out for him to come and rescue me. And he never came.'

He remembers a night when he had nothing left to give: 'I was at the end of my physical and mental and spiritual strength. It was late. It was black everywhere. I had no family around. The nurses were probably locked away in the station, but to me they weren't there. I was lying on top of my bed. The world was so black that I firmly believed, knew in my mind, that I was the only single human being left anywhere.'

He felt himself to be on the edge of a precipice. One more step and he would fall into the abyss.

He prayed that night. 'There was this coming to terms with my biological father and my heavenly Father,' he says. It was a significant moment because as he prayed he felt a response. 'There was no clap of thunder or big hand come through the ceiling. But I felt this very deep inner voice saying: *this is the worst it will get.*'

James kept his Bible with him on the ward. It was a constant at his side. He read it over and over. He often took it outside with him to let the wind flip at the pages, choosing a passage for him to read. The wind was God's breath; the passages always held a personal significance. There was another patient on the ward, an older lady who walked around in her dressing gown, shouting about the Lamb of God. James knew she was referring to him. It all tied together. He had been to Sandhurst, was a trained soldier. Trained as someone who could take life but also save it. He was going to be the judge of the quick and the dead. He was the second coming, a messianic figure, the most important person on earth.

Schizoaffective disorder

The medication James was given on the ward – those little plastic cups of orange syrup – was chlorpromazine; the first antipsychotic medicine to be developed, and known as much for its crippling side effects as for its efficacy.

He realised early on that compliance was a big issue for the staff and if he wanted to get out he'd need to take it. But he remains unconvinced that it helped all that much. 'I got well enough to come out, to be discharged. But that doesn't mean that all your thoughts that you have in hospital go away,' he explains. 'On balance, I think the side effects far outweighed its usefulness.' After a month or more he simply started to tell the psychiatrists and nurses what he figured they wanted to hear. 'That's how you often get out of hospital. Not because you're well or cured or not thinking those thoughts any more. You just say whatever you feel they're going to believe to let you out.'

He was eventually released back to his mum's house with a diagnosis of paranoid schizophrenia. In subsequent admissions this would be reviewed and changed to schizoaffective disorder: a term describing a combination of experiences associated with schizophrenia alongside those more often associated with mood disorders, such as mania and depression. More recently his diagnosis has been changed again, to bipolar disorder.

For his part, James doesn't place too much stock in the labels. He shrugs. 'I've got James syndrome.'

Feet on the ground

You realise that none of it's really true.

You were led to believe that you were someone who had great importance to the world. And then you see it was a trick. Your brain played a horrible trick on you. You feel cheated.

In time, the reality of James's situation eroded what a mental health professional might call his more *grandiose beliefs*. After leaving hospital he spent a long period slumped on his mum's sofa, staring at the TV, trying to work out where it had all gone wrong.

Every couple of weeks a community psychiatric nurse arrived to inject him with more medication. This was kept in small glass vials in his mum's fridge. Before the nurse arrived James would drag himself into the kitchen and place a vial on the Rayburn to warm it up so that the liquid would thin and hurt less going in.

On his sofa today, James reaches for his tobacco, rolls himself a cigarette. He clears his throat.

'I found it very difficult to come to terms with the fact that I failed at the army. I probably found that harder to come to terms with than that I'd developed a mental health problem. I was trying so hard to be the best and I think that makes it harder to deal with the abandonment, doesn't it? If you put everything into it. It makes it harder to come to terms with that you've been dropped like a stone and put in the guard room and told to wait for your mother. I think maybe there was a part of me that couldn't face that I'd been abandoned by the army, that I'd been rejected and kicked out. So rather than face that, I constructed this reality in my own mind that said, *No, no, you're still very important to them*.'

It wasn't easy for James to stand up from his mum's sofa and rebuild his life, and there were false starts when he tried.

More suffering. More stints in hospital.

He was told then that he shouldn't expect to ever hold down a job, have a relationship or live independently. He took that as a challenge. Ultimately James believes he has a lot to thank the army for. That if he's made a modicum of success of life, it's largely down to the fact the army taught him important skills of self-discipline and self-confidence from a very early age.

He was twenty-five when he applied to join the Devon Fire and Rescue Service. He passed the physical straight away, but reviewing his application, his full disclosure about his condition and that he'd been sectioned multiple times, the doctor in the occupational health department suggested he leave it a month or so, see how things were going, then come back. James wasn't surprised but neither was he deterred. The same thing happened four more times. James kept coming back. Word on the grapevine was that permission had to be sought from the Home Office; that James became the first retained firefighter with a known schizophrenia diagnosis.

He never got the Sword of Honour but during his eight years in the Fire Service he received a Chief Fire Officer's Commendation along with the rest of his crew for their role in a complicated rescue operation.

James is now a sought-after motivational speaker who shares his experiences to reduce discrimination and improve service provision. It's easy enough to imagine. He's a natural raconteur. He also provides consultancy and training on mental health recovery methods. When doing this, he acknowledges that his own experiences only constitute one half of his story. When he received his award from the Fire Service, his new wife, Lesley, watched on from the assembled crowd.

They met shortly after he was first unwell. Lesley's been supporting him through the turbulence in all the twenty-eight years since. A few years back, James recalls, they attended an event in Dublin together, where he was giving a talk for World Mental Health Day. He focused his lecture on the crucial role of family and carers, and after he finished the queue that formed was of people wishing to speak with his wife. She was invited onto the stage to say a few words herself, but it doesn't surprise me to hear that she declined. During my time in their home, she's opted to let James be the public speaker. For him, the important thing is knowing she's there. 'People talk about independence,' he says. 'No wonder lads in hospital are scared of leaving if they're being told it's all about independence. I don't think it is. Teach them about interdependence.'

The whole time we've been talking James's dog – a Nova Scotia Duck Tolling Retriever who goes by the name of Ella – has been curled up on the sofa beside him. She's asleep now. He rubs at her tummy. 'It's like you, Ella. You depend on us and we depend on you.'

Relapses are a part of James's life. Each time he gets unwell he's singled out, special, important. He's a soldier, a king, the Messiah. It's a long way to fall but with the unwavering support of Lesley, some close friends and a cherished dog, the landing, at least, is easier.

Diagnosis

I'VE BEEN THINKING A LOT about something James told me. About how after receiving a number of different psychiatric diagnoses, including various subtypes of schizophrenia and more recently bipolar disorder, he no longer placed too much stock in them. Enough was enough.

'I've got James Syndrome,' he'd concluded.

His experience of accumulating psychiatric labels will come as no great shock to anyone who has spent any amount of time moving through mental health services. Most of the people you will meet in this book have received at least two or three.

Of course there might be very good and legitimate reasons for a person to receive a different diagnosis at different times. If I went to my GP surgery today complaining of a painful shoulder* and then went back again next week with a nasty sore throat,† the doctor would quite rightly arrive at different explanations. So to defend the reclassifying of a person's psychiatric diagnosis over time, we might argue that it necessarily kept changing because the presenting problem kept changing. Only here's the thing: nobody (not even the staunchest defenders of psychiatry's diagnostic systems) honestly believes that this explains what's going on. In fact, a resounding failure to deliver consistently reliable diagnoses has for a long time represented something of an existential crisis for psychiatry; an Achilles' heel that its critics waste no opportunity to

---

* Which I do have, incidentally. I'm just being incredibly brave about it.
† I mention it because I can feel one coming on, though I'm not the sort to complain.

exploit. It may yet prove to be the case that 'James Syndrome' is a more sensible diagnosis than 'schizophrenia', and certainly no less scientific. I'm mindful that that's quite a claim. To begin to make sense of it we need to turn our attention for a short while to the story behind a hefty and controversial book called the *Diagnostic and Statistical Manual of Mental Disorders*, often abbreviated to DSM and commonly referred to as 'psychiatry's bible'.*

First published in 1952 by the American Psychiatric Association, the DSM was an attempt at creating a comprehensive diagnostic guidebook. It contained every mental health disorder that a person might feasibly be diagnosed with, each defined by observable symptoms that would allow the clinician to arrive at a formal diagnosis, confident in the knowledge that another doctor in possession of the *same* manual should reliably arrive at the same diagnosis. And that was the whole point of it. It was intended to finally put to rest the acknowledged problem that psychiatrists could rarely seem to agree on what was 'wrong' with their patients.

As it happened, the first edition of the DSM did little to shift this predicament. Neither did its sequel, the DSM-II, published in 1968. For both editions, the definitions of the various mental disorders were too brief and too vague to have much of an impact.

Research conducted at the time drove this problem home, revealing that two different psychiatrists seeing the same patient – sometimes mere minutes apart – would arrive at a shared diagnosis only around 50 per cent of the time.[1] It felt an awful lot like a coin flip. Educated guesswork at best. Further research emerging in the early 1970s uncovered embarrassing discrepancies in how psychiatric diagnoses were arrived at internationally. In one semi-

---

* And so, much like Holy Scripture, should be taken with a pinch of salt.

nal study a number of video recordings of mental health patients from the United States and Great Britain were shown to groups of American and British psychiatrists. The British psychiatrists concluded that they were seeing a mix of manic depressive disorders, schizophrenia and personality disorder. Their American counterparts arrived at a schizophrenia diagnosis for everyone.[2]

So psychiatric diagnostics was already on its knees (with American psychiatrists in particular gaining a reputation for a seriously trigger-happy approach to schizophrenia) when it was delivered an audacious sucker punch.

In January 1973, the psychologist David L. Rosenhan published the results of what would prove to be one of the most influential experiments in the modern history of mental healthcare. Rosenhan revealed that he and several fellow researchers had got themselves deliberately confined to mental hospitals across the United States. They did this by faking a single symptom of psychosis. Each of the researchers complained that they could hear voices, and that the voices were saying: 'Empty', 'Dull' and 'Thud'. After they were admitted to the wards they never mentioned these voices again, and instead behaved perfectly normally (whatever exactly that means). The question was: Would anyone detect that they were sane? The answer was: Nope, nobody did.[3] Astonishingly, the staff at the hospitals kept all of these 'patients' detained, in some cases for many months, insisting that they comply with medication regimes and accept they were mentally ill.

All were diagnosed with 'schizophrenia in remission' before they were released.

This experiment is sometimes offered up as evidence of cruelty or incompetence on the part of the hospital staff, perhaps partly because of its arrival in the public consciousness at around the same time as the film *One Flew Over the Cuckoo's Nest*.

People feared – albeit with a certain voyeuristic relish – that if they entered a lunatic asylum they would never get out, that they might be sane in an insane place and have Nurse Ratched to contend with. For his part, Rosenhan counselled against these more grisly interpretations:

> It could be a mistake, and a very unfortunate one, to consider that what happened to us derived from malice or stupidity on the part of the staff. Quite the contrary, our overwhelming impression of them was of people who really cared, who were committed and who were uncommonly intelligent. Where they failed, as they sometimes did painfully, it would be more accurate to attribute those failures to the environment in which they, too, found themselves than to personal callousness. Their perceptions and behavior were controlled by the situation, rather than being motivated by a malicious disposition. In a more benign environment, one that was less attached to global diagnosis, their behaviors and judgments might have been more benign and effective.[4]

Despite this caveat, it was a humiliation for American psychiatry, with reverberations felt around the world. Attacked from all sides and dissatisfied with the first two editions of the DSM, the American Psychiatric Association responded by assembling a task force whose efforts would result in the eventual publication in 1980 of DSM-III.

Okay – so possibly not the most radical response at first glance. Yet never before or since has the third instalment of a franchise proved to be quite such a game changer. This was the moment when psychiatry, or more specifically the biomedical interpretation of psychiatry, was to rise as a phoenix from the ashes and decisively stake its claim to the human mind.

In retrospect, it's hard to understand how such a significant shift came about. Reliability of clinical psychiatric diagnoses remained (and still remains) indisputably problematic.* However, DSM-III offered something that was evidently extremely powerful: a veneer of *science*. Gone was all the woolly Freudian and psychoanalytical vernacular that the profession had for so long been enamoured of. It was replaced now with detailed, explicit and highly specific diagnostic criteria for each of its disorders, complete with easy-to-read tables and lists.

Take depression, for example. DSM-II called this 'depressive neurosis' and described it as 'manifested by an excessive reaction of depression due to an internal conflict or to an identifiable event such as the loss of a love object or cherished possession'.[5] In contrast, the definition of the newly coined 'major depression' in DSM-III ran over several pages, including a checklist. To meet the criteria the patient would need to experience at least five discrete symptoms. One of these would be a dysphoric mood, along with four others from a list of eight, including poor appetite, insomnia, loss of energy, suicidality and so on.[6] These symptoms would need to present nearly every day for a period of at least two weeks. There were also detailed exclusion criteria. It's all extremely precise; a

---

* It's worth mentioning here that the American-produced DSM is not the only classification tool for diagnosing mental disorders. The World Health Organisation has its own similar taxonomy, called the *International Classification of Disorders* (ICD). This was already on its ninth revision when DSM-III was released. However, DSM-III was shown to be used and preferred over the ICD-9 by psychiatrists and mental health professionals worldwide, hence my emphasis on it. In the UK today, it's not uncommon for clinicians to refer to both systems or neither, which in some ways is a practical stance, though it certainly can't improve diagnostic reliability.

common language to describe exactly what depression is and what it is not. Same for manic depression. Same for schizophrenia.

On the face of it that might all seem eminently sensible. Just as it was eminently sensible – indeed, necessary – that in 1974 (for the sixth printing of DSM-II) homosexuality was finally removed from the official list of diagnosable mental disorders.

What we need to ask, though, is how these decisions are made. Why is depression composed of five symptoms rather than four or six? Why must they be present for two weeks rather than two days or two months? Why is homosexuality a mental illness in 1973 and not a mental illness in 1974?

These are good questions because they lead us to an important criticism of the DSM, and by extension reveal a weakness in the very foundations upon which psychiatry is constructed.

'The way I sometimes explain it is that back in the sixteenth century a group of villagers could probably reliably agree that their neighbour was a witch.' This is the clinical psychologist and author Dr Lucy Johnstone again. You'll remember we met her earlier when thinking about stigma. She argues that the quickest and easiest way to get rid of mental health stigma would be to get rid of mental health diagnoses. Much like James, she doesn't place too much stock in the names of these things. In fact, she doesn't believe they're things at all. 'There was once a great trend of identifying witches,' she explains. 'It would probably have been the case that everybody in the village would reliably identify that the old lady who lived on the edge of the village with her cats and her broomstick was a witch. So a reliable judgement. But does that mean they genuinely identified a witch?'

Lucy Johnstone is talking about the difference between the scientific concepts of 'reliability' (which refers to the extent to which assessments are consistent) and 'validity' (meaning, at its simplest, how well this reflects an objective reality). 'So you might be able to get everybody to agree that a person has schizophrenia,' Johnstone continues, 'although in practice it seems impossible to do even that. But suppose you did, does that mean you've identified something real? The DSM only aims for reliability, not validity. We have no idea at all whether these diagnoses meaningfully relate to anything in the real world. In my view, they don't.'

Our instinct might be to balk at this. Terms such as depression, ADHD and schizophrenia are used ubiquitously and without so much as a hint of interrogation across all sectors of the media and in our daily lives. How can they not relate to something in the real world?

More specifically, how can they not relate to that small part of the real world that is our brain or genetic material?

Needless to say, psychiatric diagnoses get a fair bit of airtime in psychiatric hospitals. When I was working as a nurse, during clinical handovers (when information about patients is discussed within the team) a person's diagnosis would frequently be the first thing mentioned about them, alongside their name and section status under the Mental Health Act: 'Mohammed X, section 3, a long history of paranoid schizophrenia . . .' 'Jane Y, informal, looks like a first presentation of bipolar . . .' and so on.

To be clear, I'm not suggesting that their diagnosis was the *whole* of the clinical handover. It was not. A good deal of time would also be spent discussing in detail how the people under our care reported that they were feeling, along with other observations relating to care plans, risk assessments, medication reviews and the like. But certainly a person's diagnosis holds a highly prominent position within all this, declared right at the start, as real and concrete as their name. That couldn't mean nothing, right?

To help unpick these questions, Lucy Johnstone highlights an important distinction between the *symptoms* and *signs* of medical conditions.[7]

Symptoms are the complaints that a person might take along to their doctor or pharmacist, such as nausea, pain or fatigue. Often these are entirely subjective in nature. Let's imagine, for example, that someone goes to their GP because they are feeling thirsty all of the time, despite drinking plenty of water. That's a subjective symptom, insofar as there's no way for the GP to confirm or verify the patient's feeling of thirst. Instead, she would take this patient at their word and start to think about possible causes.

She might ask if the patient is experiencing anything else out of the ordinary. And let's say that this patient is indeed experiencing other symptoms: they're tired a lot of the time, and come to think of it, they've lost a bit of weight recently. At this point (because the GP knows that she exists only within an explanatory vignette in a book about 'mental illness' and so understands implicitly that there is only one possible comparator we're driving towards here) diabetes might be suspected.

But such a diagnosis would not be made *only* on the basis of these subjective symptoms. Instead, the GP would seek to confirm her suspicions by testing for an underlying sign – the difference being that unlike many symptoms, signs can be observed and confirmed by others, and can be compared to an objective standard or norm.

So in this case, a sign that might begin to confirm the diagnosis of diabetes is raised glucose levels, as objectively verifiable by tests.

Crucially, the biological connection between this sign and the patient's described symptoms is well understood. The raised blood glucose levels are the result of poor cellular absorption and increased excretion of glucose. This in turn means that the body must burn more of its fat and muscle reserves for energy – hence the fatigue and weight loss.

That's not to say diabetes is fully understood. As with most medical conditions, our understanding of it is evolving all the time, and in recent years different discrete biological causes for these abnormal glucose levels (signs of the signs, we might say) have been discovered, which in turn are leading us towards more tailored treatment options. Notwithstanding that, it's this process of connecting the symptoms of a condition with their underlying biological causes that forms the bedrock of clinical diagnostics in *all branches of medicine* with the single exception of psychiatry.

'I don't think it's widely appreciated,' says Dr Lucy Johnstone, 'that there's no solid evidence at all that these psychiatric problems – the vast majority of them anyway – are the result of identifiable causes in the body or brain.'

It's true to say that in my many years of working on psychiatric wards, and accepting with complete confidence that Mohammed X *had* paranoid schizophrenia and Jane Y *had* bipolar, never did I once pop down to the clinic with Mohammed or Jane to arrange for them to have a brain scan or blood test to confirm these diagnoses.

Never. Not once.

We can't. Such tests do not exist.* And it's this missing piece of the jigsaw that renders the science behind psychiatric diagnostics more than a little bit questionable.

Upon publication in 2013 of the latest edition of the *Diagnostic and Statistical Manual* – DSM-5 – Thomas Insel, the director of the US National Institute of Mental Health (the world's largest mental health research organisation) wrote:

> The goal of this new manual, as with all previous editions, is to provide a common language for describing psychopathology. While DSM has been described as a 'Bible' for the field, it is, at best, a dictionary, creating a set of labels and defining each. The strength of each of the editions of DSM has been 'reliability' – each edition has ensured that

---

* Or rather, they don't exist for the overwhelming majority of psychiatric disorders. There is a small minority that can absolutely be tested for in such a way. Many forms of dementia can be clearly observed in brain scans and there is a genetic test to confirm a diagnosis of Huntington's disease. These along with a smattering of other such neurological conditions are often collectively described as the 'organic' mental disorders precisely because of their observable organic aetiology. However, most of the DSM (and ICD) psychiatric diagnoses, including so-called schizophrenia, so-called bipolar, so-called clinical depression, so-called borderline personality disorder (BPD), so-called obsessive–compulsive disorder (OCD), so-called generalised anxiety disorder (GAD), so-called eating disorders, so-called post-traumatic stress disorder (PTSD), so-called attention deficit hyperactivity disorder (ADHD), so-called body dysmorphic disorder, so-called delusional disorder, so-called dependent personality disorder, so-called cyclothymia, so-called disinhibited social engagement disorder, so-called dissociative identity disorder (DID), so-called skin-picking disorder, so-called exhibitionistic disorder, so-called factitious disorder, so-called transvestic disorder, so-called fetishistic disorder, so-called frotteuristic disorder, so-called hoarding disorder, so-called nightmare disorder, so-called illness anxiety disorder, so-called intermittent explosive disorder, so-called panic disorder, so-called rumination disorder, so-called hypoactive sexual desire disorder, so-called narcissistic personality disorder, so-called social anxiety disorder and many, many more, have no comprehensively proven biological cause and there exist no objectively verifiable tests for them.

clinicians use the same terms in the same ways. The weakness is its lack of validity . . . Patients with mental disorders deserve better.[8]

Faced with this and a barrage of similar criticism from voices across the professional spectrum, the chair of the DSM-5 committee, Dr David Kupfer, conceded:

In the future, we hope to be able to identify disorders using biological and genetic markers that provide precise diagnoses that can be delivered with complete reliability and validity. Yet this promise, which we have anticipated since the 1970s, remains disappointingly distant. We've been telling patients for several decades that we are waiting for biomarkers. We're still waiting.[9]

All this raises an important question. If psychiatric diagnoses aren't informed by objectively verifiable underlying biological signs then what exactly does inform them? We can now also return to the questions that I asked earlier: Why is homosexuality a mental illness one year and not the next? And how have psychiatric diagnostic criteria, at least since DSM-III, become so very specific?

The short answer (which is also the long answer) is that we make it up as we go along.

Or at least, groups of influential psychiatrists do. The groundbreaking DSM-III was a team effort, chaired by a psychiatrist named Dr Robert Spitzer who assembled a group of ideologically like-minded colleagues to set about deleting from and, mostly, adding to the disorders outlined in DSM-II, as well as agreeing on their definitions and diagnostic criteria.*

Put another way, what we confidently call the mental illnesses are decided by committee.

These committees, and the people they consult with, will be rightly influenced by what they have observed in clinical practice, but they will also be influenced by other forces – political, social and economic. That's why homosexuality stopped being a mental illness: the times they were a-changin'. And it was the voice of feminism that narrowly won the argument against 'premenstrual syndrome' and 'masochistic personality disorder' (read: the domestic violence you're suffering is your own fault) finding their way into the 1987 DSM-III-Revised.[10]

In an interview in 2007, the psychiatrist and author Daniel J. Carlat asked Dr Spitzer how exactly he and his team arrived at the decision that a person would need to be experiencing a minimum of five separate symptoms to warrant a diagnosis of major depression. Spitzer smiled impishly and replied, 'Because four just seemed like not enough. And six seemed like too much.'[11]

Now, we might intuitively agree with all of that. *Of course* homosexuality isn't a disorder. It should never have been categorised as a disorder in the first place. And five is a very nice, complete sort of number.

What we mustn't do, though, is confuse any of this with science.

---

* Spitzer and his colleagues were known as the neo-Kraepelinians. Emil Kraepelin was mentioned earlier in this book as the physician who first described schizophrenia. Considered by many to be the founder of modern psychiatry, he arrived on the scene at around the same time as Sigmund Freud, and in many ways was his ideological opposite. Kraepelin believed firmly that mental illness was the result of biological aberrations and devoted much of his career to developing a psychiatric taxonomy. The psychoanalytically trained psychiatrists of the 1950s and 60s largely eschewed these ideas, believing diagnosis to be an impediment to therapy. Spitzer and his fellow neo-Kraepelinians were therefore something of a fringe group until they completely stole the show with DSM-III.

The DSM is – in the words of another former director of the National Institute of Mental Health, Dr Steven Hyman – 'an absolute scientific nightmare'.[12]

For all of that, it would be wrong to characterise mental health diagnoses as completely arbitrary. They're not. They are the names given to clusters of human experiences that have been observed to frequently group together.

A young child in a classroom who often seems to have difficulty in keeping her attention on what the teacher is saying might also be easily distracted by things going on around her. She mightn't seem to listen to instructions. She might have difficulty waiting her turn and so interrupt the other children while fidgeting restlessly in her seat. Such behaviours are seen together often enough that there emerges from them the 'mental illness' of ADHD. And so it goes for virtually every other diagnosis. A terrified adolescent who claims to hear voices telling him to hurt himself might well also have distressing and strange thoughts. He's being persecuted by his neighbours. He's having ideas inserted into his mind with telepathy. He's withdrawn socially, appears flat in mood, and his parents claim he's lost all initiative in life. Such a story is seen often enough that there emerges a pattern, a notion, an idea – and we call this idea schizophrenia.

A spanner in the diagnostic works is that many of these patterns of human experiences have rather blurred edges. A person who experiences some of the typical thoughts of so-called schizophrenia may also be experiencing many of the feelings associated with so-called depression or bipolar. This partly explains why so many psychiatric patients end up with so many different labels, and also goes some way towards explaining a staggering proliferation over the decades in the number of official psychiatric disorders that are said to exist. The DSM-I outlined 128 mental health disorders that you or I might be found to be suffering from. DSM-III added a hundred or so more and the trend has continued. DSM-5 lists 541.

Something looks a bit like schizophrenia and a bit like bipolar? *Et voilà*: schizoaffective disorder.

Or if someone is experiencing a quality of suffering that exhibits some of the hallmarks of an existing diagnosis but falls a little shy of it in intensity, that's okay, they're allowed to have a medical-sounding illness too. Not quite clinically depressed? That's dysthymia. Not quite bipolar? That's cyclothymia. To borrow the phrase used by many critics of mental health diagnostics: there's a disorder for everyone. The influence of pharmaceutical companies will have played its part in this phenomenon. Many academics also suggest it's no coincidence that this process started in the 1980s under Thatcher in the UK and Reagan in the US, with the rise of a neo-liberal agenda that began redefining citizens as consumers and characterising poverty as the fault of the poor.

We know that extreme poverty and social inequality have a negative impact on our mental wellbeing, and there's no doubt that this has become entangled with politics. The proliferation of the psychiatric disorders may – at least to some degree – serve the interests of people in positions of political power. Better it be understood that a young millennial who's falling apart while struggling to pay two thirds of their increasingly precarious salary to rent a mouldy room in a shared house is suffering from a 'panic disorder' than countenance the possibility that the real sickness is located elsewhere.

Today, psychiatric diagnoses can feel not entirely dissimilar to brands – with the currently more 'popular brands'* such as

---

* I'm not suggesting that these are popular in the sense of being *desirable* to those who suffer from them; simply that more public attention, empathy and resources go their way.

'depression' and 'anxiety' getting marketed and monetised to a far greater extent, resulting in the publication of huge numbers of self-help books and the development of new therapies, while less marketable brands such as the so-called personality disorders suffer from a diminished investment – and so yet another inequity is forged.

Personally, I reckon Stephen Fry was on to something when he observed that 'labelling reveals more about the state of society than the state of the human mind'. (He was referring to his own experiences of being diagnosed with both cyclothymia and bipolar, concluding, rather poetically, that 'a butterfly will flutter by just the same whether you call it a pretty creature, a Monarch or *Danaus plexippus*. Naming is important but can sometimes block rather than aid comprehension.*)

Dr Lucy Johnstone and others argue that beyond the unscientific methods of mental health diagnoses there is the additional problem that their described 'symptoms' consist predominantly of a person's thoughts, feelings and behaviours, and for such things it can be extremely difficult to determine where to draw the line between what's 'normal' and what's 'abnormal'. Even highly skilled clinicians can (and often do) come to different conclusions about

---

* This quote is taken from a foreword that Fry contributed to *Taming the Beast Within: Shredding the Stereotypes of Personality Disorder* by Professor Peter Tyrer. Upon its publication in 2018 this book was immediately given brutally scathing reviews by large numbers of people who took exception to its poorly considered title, which they argued would only serve to propagate rather than challenge stereotypes. It's a reasonable point. It's well known that many people – though certainly not all – who end up with a personality disorder diagnosis have suffered pretty horrendous childhoods, often involving physical, emotional or sexual abuse. To suggest that the 'beast' is somehow a part of the sufferer rather than a cruelty they've endured was always going to cause upset and anger. At the same time, I don't imagine for one second that this was the author's intention. He was probably trying to help people. As I've said already, there's no uncontroversial language when talking about these things. If in doubt, though, best not to evoke beasts.

what constitutes a child's 'appropriate' level of attention in order to arrive at a diagnosis of ADHD, for instance.

Our thoughts and feelings are already highly subjective experiences, to which mental health professionals must then bring another layer of subjective judgement. As the consultant child and adolescent psychiatrist Sami Timimi describes it:

> When a clinician claims that a patient is clinically depressed, or has ADHD, or has bipolar disorder, or whatever, not only is he trying to turn something based on subjective opinion into something that appears scientific, but he is also reifying the event – turning something subjective into something 'concrete'. This causes a kind of 'tunnel vision' where the psychiatric diagnostic version of events becomes the dominant story and alternative ways of viewing the situation are pushed to one side. Hence, if someone believes ADHD is a 'real' disorder that exists in the brain and is potentially lifelong, that person – and those who know them – may come to act according to this belief. This is to create a pessimistic self-fulfilling prophecy.[13]

There can be no greater risk of this than for so-called schizophrenia. 'As soon as you say it's schizophrenia we stop looking,' says Johnstone. 'We've got a pseudo-explanation which stops us looking any further. It's no longer professionally, scientifically or ethically acceptable to present these diagnoses as if they are undisputed fact.'

It's an argument I take to the psychiatrist Professor Sir Robin Murray, widely considered to be the UK's pre-eminent schizophrenia researcher. We'll turn to his research in due course, but on the single issue of diagnosis he's unequivocal: 'Although I've spent a lifetime doing research into schizophrenia,' he tells me, 'I don't believe it exists as a discrete entity. I wouldn't say to patients that they have schizophrenia. It's such an insult in many ways. I'm more likely to say that they have a vulnerability to what psychiatrists call psychosis.' This view of schizophrenia as the extreme end of a psychosis spectrum as opposed to a categorical illness in its own right is shared by many of the mental health clinicians and researchers that I've worked with. This may be because I'm British. As was the case prior to DSM-III, there remains a significant divide between European and American interpretations, and in the United States the view of schizophrenia as a deteriorating brain disease (not unlike dementia) is still prevalent, despite having been, according to Professor Murray, fatally undermined by the evidence. In a recent article he wrote: 'The syndrome is already beginning to break down, for example into those cases caused by copy number variations, drug abuse, social adversity, etc. Presumably this process will accelerate, and the term schizophrenia will be confined to history, like "dropsy".'[14] Unsurprisingly, he's highly sceptical of the DSM, dismissing it as a parochial American system that's nothing to do with us.

So why, I ask, do its categories continue to be the bedrock of so much clinical discussion and research, even in the UK?

His answer strikes me as both honest and shocking: 'It is true that researchers like myself, we often have to use DSM criteria in our research papers,' he acknowledges. 'And the reason for that is our publications have got to get into American journals because your survival in the university system depends on your impact factor. And your h-index.* And getting a paper in the *American Journal of Psychiatry* is worth three times as much as getting it in

---

* The h-index is a kind of academic footprint that measures how many papers a researcher publishes and how many times these papers get cited in other papers.

the *British Journal of Psychiatry*. So we would sometimes use these criteria even though we don't necessarily believe in them.'

It's a depressing view that's echoed by other scientists I've spoken with. Even among those who are less concerned about being published in US scientific journals there's still a sense of frustration that their hands are tied. The general consensus goes something like this: *There's no doubt that categorical diagnoses (such as depression and schizophrenia) are misleading to patients. And that they get in the way of research. But the whole industry of clinical study design rests on them, so what can we do?* The dilemma is that in order to conduct research, participants need to be recruited. Clearly this recruitment needs to be based on something and invariably that's a pre-existing diagnosis. It's a vicious circle. As one senior researcher told me: 'If a DSM or similar such diagnosis is the requirement to enter into a study, if that study is then positive and proves the beneficial effects of your intervention, well, that intervention will only be applicable to other people with the same unscientific diagnosis. We're constraining our own advances.'

And yet our advances do creep forwards. As we will discover, there are many credible theories about what causes people to have the kind of experiences we currently call schizophrenia, and from these we can be hopeful there will emerge more effective ways to alleviate suffering.

For all the debate about the reality behind diagnosis, there can be no uncertainty about the reality of people's pain – and sometimes, tragically, this pain is unbearable.

THE MOTHER

Different ways of dying

TEN-YEAR-OLD JOE is lying on his back on the kitchen floor. His eyes are closed. His head is turned at a slight angle. The thick tangles of his blond hair have come to rest beside the plastic feet of a children's easel.

From this photograph I can't make out the blade of the knife, but it appears to have plunged deep into the side of his neck.

'He was always a practical joker,' Clare says. She's showing me an album on Facebook, with maybe twenty or thirty pictures of Joe. But the timeline's all muddled up, so we flip back and forth from images of an alert, bright, boundlessly energetic little boy, showing off his skateboard or playing with his younger brother and sister at their home in New Haven, Connecticut, to pictures of Joe as a teenager, seventeen or eighteen years old, on day release from various psychiatric units in Cardiff, Wales.

In one of these the family have gathered in Roath Park, a popular Victorian park in central Cardiff. It's a bright, cold Christmas morning and they're beside the lake. Clare is there, along with Joe's stepfather, Ed, and their other children. Joe's little sister is clambering onto her new bike. A grandparent is wearing a paper hat from a Christmas cracker. Joe's standing a little to the side of everyone, at the edge of the frame. His curly blond locks have been shaved away. He's grown extremely heavy. His face is pale and puffy. His expression – as he looks towards the camera – is completely blank.

Then a swipe of the screen and we're with the exuberant little boy again: a boy who loved slapstick comedy and Mr Bean and wildlife and dinosaurs, and who in this picture is attempting to acrobatically scale the inside of a doorframe. It's difficult to reconcile the two images; to see the same person, separated by such a short stretch of time. 'He went from a beautiful boy to—' Clare lowers her voice. She searches for the right words. 'Sometimes I found it hard to look at him.'

Less than ten years after Joe played at being dead on the kitchen floor of a bustling family home in New Haven, he would die, all alone, in a dirty flat in Cardiff, never to find the sandwiches that Clare had placed outside his door, worried that her son might be hungry.

There are different kinds of parental grief and it's possible to feel jealous of the circumstances that surround other children's deaths. This is something Clare teaches me. It is possible to see news footage of young soldiers who have been killed in Iraq, returned to their parents in coffins draped with Union flags, and to desperately try to push away a feeling of envy because those parents can be proud of how their sons died.

It's possible to be jealous of the mother whose child's life was cut short by leukaemia. *What a wonderful child, what a tragic loss. What a socially acceptable way to die.*

It is possible to ache with guilt for having such thoughts. For this guilt to drain your energy, to send you to your bed. To compound your own messy and horrible and shameful kind of grief. Grief suffered alone.

Clare and I have found a bench in Roath Park, a short walk from where the family photograph was taken.

It was Clare's suggestion that we meet here. The park is close to the last house that Joe lived in with the whole family before everything unravelled. Many of Clare's memories feel stitched into physical locations, and during our time together she takes me to some of the places where these memories are kept.

I have the sense that I've met Clare at a turning point in her life. Eight years after the death of her eldest son, she's recently divorced and figuring out what she wants to do with her future. She used to be a physicist. She gained her PhD at the University of Cambridge. But she's reluctant to share details of her career, and moreover seems vaguely suspicious of my reasons for wanting to include even these few brief details as a backdrop to her story.

The problem, she explains to me, in a soft Scottish accent that she's kept from her childhood in Ayrshire, is that it's a kind of short-hand. By including such biographical details what I'm actually say-ing is: *Meet Clare. Look how educated and clever and middle-class she is. She can't be a bad mum. None of this is her fault.*

Clare isn't comfortable with that.

High expectations

Joe was a mistake. Clare never meant to get pregnant. Mark – his biological father – was fun to spend time with, at least at the begin-ning, but in Clare's words 'definitely wasn't husband material'.

It was a brief, tumultuous relationship that ended acrimoniously, and so at twenty-three, still completing her PhD, Clare found herself a single mum raising a little boy.

She met Ed, a neuroscientist, when Joe was one year old. They became a family and five years later Clare and Ed had their first child together, another little boy whom they named Jack. Clare recalls how Ed was absolutely besotted with Jack, his first child. Sometimes the contrast in his affection for the two boys was difficult for Clare to deal with, even if she could rationalise it. She believes Ed worked hard in his relationship with Joe but the parental bond perhaps wasn't ever quite there. It mightn't have helped that Joe was so boisterous, whereas Jack was quieter, more introverted, more content in his own company – in short, more like his dad.

Jack was two years old and Joe was coming up to eight when Clare and Ed made the decision to move to the United States. This was a career opportunity for Ed – a lectureship at Yale University.

Clare became a stay-at-home mum to the two boys. Initially this arrangement was intended to be only for one year, then Clare would pick up with her own career again. That's how she reconciled herself to the decision, though deep down she also felt relieved. She'd been struggling to balance the pressures of her career with the pressures of being a mum. She was stressed and tired, and this new arrangement felt like a way of saving face. It wasn't: 'This is too much. I'm going to give up my career.' It was: 'Oh, we're going to focus on my husband's career for a bit.' Then two years after moving to the States their daughter, Lucy, was born, and Clare's unexpected new life as a mother and housewife was fully cemented.

It was, at least for a short while, a nice and comfortable sort of life. A life of settling into an exciting new culture and listening with adoring amusement as her children developed their American accents. Clare recollects a favourite family video of her daughter at nursery school, with her pudgy little hand pressed against her heart as she pledges allegiance to the flag.

She recalls the garage door of their new home in one of New Haven's affluent, leafy neighbourhoods. It was electric, remote-controlled, and at the time seemed somehow to epitomise the whole American way of life. A life of play dates for the kids and dinner parties for the adults, all within a privileged community of extremely high achievers with the highest of expectations. That's not to say there were no difficulties whatsoever. When Joe was nine or ten it became clear that he was struggling academically. He couldn't grasp some fairly basic maths concepts and the teachers at his school asked that he be tested for ADHD. This was the late 1990s when testing and treatment for the condition was rife across much of the US.* He ticked a few of the boxes but not enough to get a diagnosis, and certainly not enough for Clare to consider stuffing him full of Ritalin in order to calm him down in the classroom (which she suspected was what they really wanted). Being British, they weren't about to go down that route.

Then Joe hit adolescence.

Down towards zero

They tried grounding him and confiscating his beloved computer games, along with positive reinforcement: 'If you behave well enough we'll have a treat, get ice cream sundaes.' The problem was

---

* In fact, this phenomenon has been directly linked to the publication of the fourth edition of the DSM in 1994, which led to a startling three-fold increase in the number of children being diagnosed with ADHD. The task force for DSM-IV was chaired by the American psychiatrist Allen Frances, who has since spoken and written extensively of his profound regret at what he calls an epidemic of this diagnosis. This has been especially visible in the United States, where by 2013 a staggering 11 per cent of children aged between four and seventeen were diagnosed as having ADHD, with huge numbers of children being prescribed (obscenely profitable) medication. Frances has argued that this over-treatment is being fuelled by irresponsible drug companies, by careless diagnosing and prescribing on the part of physicians, and by worried parents and harried teachers. He suggests that most – though, of course, not all – of what passes for ADHD is nothing more than normal variation or developmental difference, and also highlights the deeply troubling fact that the youngest child in a classroom is more than twice as likely to be diagnosed than the oldest, concluding that we've turned immaturity into a disease.

that none of it was working. Joe had no interest in ice cream sundaes. He stopped wanting to join in with family activities. At thirteen years of age, he still adored his baby sister but was withdrawing from the rest of the family. He had become a sullen figure, mildly depressed. He was getting into trouble at school.

On one occasion, he stole prescription sleeping tablets from Ed and sold them to his classmates. Another time, he got caught shoplifting cough medicine from the local pharmacy, seeking out the kind with an ingredient to get high on. Clare tried to rationalise it. He was a rebellious teenager. It would be a phase. When Joe was coming to the end of middle school, Clare attended a special assembly organised for the parents. The headteacher took to the stage and offered a few insouciant words of reassurance to everyone: 'If your kids get to high school without getting in any trouble with the police, you're probably doing okay.' In the ripple of laughter, Clare took comfort. Fine, yes, Joe had been in a bit of trouble with the police, but for stealing cough syrup. In the grand scheme of things that wasn't such a big deal.

Only things kept getting worse. By the time Joe was fourteen they couldn't leave alcohol or any money in the house as it would inevitably go missing. He was drinking excessively, smoking marijuana, bunking off school, caring less and less.

His relationship with his stepfather was completely breaking down as Ed adopted the ever more futile role of 'enforcer of the rules', to which Joe responded with undisguised hostility. Clare believes Ed's primary motivation by this time was simply protecting his own two children from the impact of Joe's behaviour. That was painful to accept, even if on some level she could understand it – and, of course, she too felt the need to shield Jack and Lucy from the destructive presence of their elder brother.

I want to know how Clare's relationship with Joe was holding up while all this was unfolding. It's a question we come back to several times.

Clare can see Joe with Ed clearly enough, recall the creeping mistrust between them, the shouting and the swearing. And she can picture Joe protectively standing over little Lucy as she pushes her toy wheelbarrow in the garden. But the moments when it was just her and Joe – they're that much harder for Clare to unearth. There's so much from this time that she has buried.

He was never aggressive towards her – she's certain of that – but neither was he affectionate. Evenings of snuggling up on the couch together to watch *The Simpsons* were a thing of the past. What few words she and Joe shared were mostly strained and loaded with conflict. She might challenge him about some money missing from her purse. He might grunt a reply: 'It wasn't me, get off my back.' Then a familiar, heavy silence would resume between them, punctuated by a slammed door and Joe barricading himself in his room.

She read all the books, learnt all the strategies – about setting clear boundaries, emphasising that her love was unconditional but that they weren't prepared to put up with his behaviour.

It was around this time that they tried a tougher kind of love. Ed removed Joe's bedroom door ('You have to earn your privacy, Joe') and took away his front door key. It had no effect whatsoever. Joe got in with a crowd of older kids – some with cars, at least one with an apartment. He disappeared for days at a time.

Clare consciously stopped socialising, in part because she was exhausted and in part because she dreaded the moment when conversations would turn to how everyone's kids were getting on. It was too painful to hear her friends proudly listing their children's achievements, or else bemoaning minor grievances about laziness and backchat, while Joe was *God knows where* and by now awaiting trial on a drugs charge.

At the same time, she didn't feel able to confide in these friends. It wasn't so long ago she'd held such high expectations for Joe; expectations that had been incrementally lowered, and were now, in Clare's words, 'down towards zero'. It all seemed too shameful, somehow. An indictment of bad parenting. She was afraid of being judged. It was easier to stay at home.

The drug offence was about as minor as they get. Joe and a friend were caught hiding in some bushes with a tiny bag of marijuana. But this was a legal system fighting hard against the city's growing drugs culture, and Clare recalls the police officer at the station making it clear that he considered Joe to be the lowest of the low. They were trying to give him a fright.

Everything began to feel more serious when the trial started. The court was in a neighbourhood with a reputation for violent crime. 'We lived in this tiny island of privilege and academia surrounded by real poverty,' Clare says. In fact, this was the subject of a bruising exposé published in *GQ* magazine around this time, which described Yale University as struggling amid 'a war zone of poverty, crime, and drugs as frightening as any American city'. Waiting on a graffiti-scrawled bench in the long corridor outside the courtrooms, Clare looked around, avoiding eye contact with those she imagined were hardened criminals, gang members, people who'd been in shootings and drug deals gone wrong. For the first time she began to contemplate the unthinkable: *What if Joe doesn't turn a corner? What if this is his future?* She shook the thought away, clinging on to the hope that this place would give her son the push he needed, that he wouldn't want to be in this position again.

The trial was over in a blur. There was a small fine to be paid and Joe was ordered to spend one week in a secure detox ward for teenagers with drug and alcohol problems, followed by mandatory weekly visits to a counselling centre for troubled adolescents.

Joe, fifteen years of age, with spots and greasy skin and long hair that he insisted on cutting himself, slumped in the dock. He wasn't bothered in the slightest. He wasn't scared. He showed no remorse. More unsettling than all of this: he looked oddly, incongruously amused.

Slipping away

Joe's behaviour was a big factor in the family deciding to return to the UK. He'd been expelled from school. He remained completely out of control. Increasingly isolated from her friends, and with constant worry and stress taking its toll on her marriage, Clare felt horribly alone. She hoped that by returning home they would be able to draw more support from family, get Joe back into education, and somehow start over again.

There were other factors, too. Clare was done with her role of '1950s-style housewife', cooking and cleaning while her husband went to work. She didn't have a work permit and this, on top of everything else, sealed the deal. Ed secured a job for himself at Cardiff University and they packed their bags.

On the morning they were due to leave, Joe was missing, off with a group of mates who frequently drove around the city to buy drugs. He was taking anything he could lay his hands on, including, Clare believes, trying heroin and crack cocaine, along with various prescription drugs and alcohol. He'd been gone for days.

Clare was frantic, felt physically sick, although it was hardly unexpected. She and Ed had even gone as far as seeking legal advice in preparation for this very eventuality. What if Joe outright refused to come back with them? Could they force him? Was it conceivable they could leave the States without him, send over money and arrange for him to fly over later? The lawyer leaned across his desk, glancing pointedly at a framed photograph of his own children. 'You've got a fifteen-year-old child,' he offered. 'And you're seriously contemplating moving continents and leaving him behind. Get a grip.'

Of course she wasn't going to leave without him. If he wasn't going then she wasn't going either. Whatever was to happen next would be entirely on Joe's terms.

There were a lot of people that Clare never said a proper good-bye to. She didn't have the emotional or mental resources to arrange a leaving party or anything remotely like one. She felt guilty for not doing that. It was the sort of thing she expected herself to do, but she couldn't put on the show. It was all she could manage to climb into the taxi to the airport (actually a stretch limo; an attempt to try to make the day feel special for Jack and Lucy) with the horrible sinking feeling of leaving under a cloud, of silently and shamefully slipping away.

Joe turned up at the house with less than an hour to spare.

Like father, like son

How did Joe feel about leaving New Haven – the place where he'd lived for most of his life? He had just turned sixteen, and though Clare didn't know or approve of his friends, he clearly still had a social life: people he was hanging out with, taking drugs with. People he might feel sad to leave behind.

Sitting on our bench in Roath Park, ignoring the first spits of rain, Clare thinks on this for a while. The truth is, they don't know how he felt. It was impossible to have that kind of conversation with him.

Joe never said that he cared about leaving. But neither did he seem to care about anything else. During his court-ordered programme of therapy in New Haven, his counsellor had noted: 'It's unusual just how little he's bothered by what's going on in his own life.'

Clare recalls an exception, though: 'He was *desperate* to hang out with his real dad.'

In the years since their acrimonious split when Joe was a baby, Clare had stayed in vague contact with Mark through his mother, who as Joe's paternal grandmother had always wanted to remain a part of his life.

Clare learnt that Mark had become very unwell in his early thirties, at some point receiving a diagnosis of paranoid schizophrenia. According to Mark's mother, medication kept him on an even keel. He was managing though certainly not thriving. He had fairly serious problems with alcohol. He'd go out on benders, use up his benefits, and because he wasn't working would then live off beans on toast until the next benefit cheque came through. Despite all this, when he heard that his son was returning to the UK, Mark reached out to him.

It's difficult today for Clare to separate the few brief conversations she had with Joe about this from the many interpretations and theories she has constructed in her own mind. But she does recall an occasion when – in a rare moment of openness – Joe confided to her that the family with his stepfather didn't feel real; that he didn't feel he belonged.

Joe figured he had more in common with the other side of his family – the side without PhDs.

A month or so after they started their new lives in Cardiff, Joe shuffled onto a coach to Cambridge in his baggy jeans and hoodie, a bag slung across his shoulder.

Clare believes Joe hoped that by spending some time with his biological dad he might find his place in life, start to work out who he was and what he wanted. Joe expected to stay for a couple of weeks. After only a couple of days Clare received a phone call.

Mark's voice sounded panicked. He told Clare he couldn't cope. It was a nightmare. All Joe wanted to do was get high and drink. He couldn't control him. He didn't know what to do.

Upon returning to Cardiff, Joe was visibly crestfallen. He'd built it all up so much. 'My own dad fucking hates me.'

That night Joe wandered out into Roath Park to sit and drink bottles of strong cider and smoke cannabis with a group of fishermen who would pitch tents along the banks of the lake and fish in the cold dark water.

It would be on an anniversary of his son's death that Mark would one day die by suicide.

If you say it quietly

It's difficult for Clare to describe it. 'He kept his transatlantic accent,' she tells me, 'his American twang. But his words slowed down. They became slurred, less animated. He sounded . . .' She hesitates. 'He sounded sort of thick.'

This change in how Joe spoke was marked and sudden and it frightened Clare. It convinced her that something was really wrong with him, that there was more going on here than rebellious teenage behaviour. There had to be. She dragged him along to a GP in Cardiff, who in turn referred him for a mental health assessment.

They sat in a small, airless room. On a low table was a box of tissues and an empty water jug. The mental health professional ('the psychiatrist or psychologist or whoever it was') asked Joe questions about his mood and thoughts and worries. *What's been on your mind recently? Do you have any beliefs that aren't shared by others you know? Have you ever felt your life was not worth living? Do you ever feel that others can hear what you're thinking? Have you ever attempted to end your life? Do you ever think about harming others?* That sort of thing.

Joe gave his answers.

Clare talked about how her son's voice had changed. But it didn't seem to tick any boxes. Besides, this person had never heard Joe speak before. Nobody in Cardiff knew him. And it wasn't as though his voice was objectively strange. Only that his mother was convinced it had changed.

Joe wasn't concerned.

Clare felt a desperate, rising frustration: 'They didn't think anything was wrong with him.'

He wasn't hearing voices, had no obviously paranoid or strange thoughts, wasn't depressed. No help was offered. Joe was left to his own devices.

Ed was adamant about what they needed to do, and even through the fog of exhaustion Clare could see his reasoning.

But that didn't mean she wanted to do it.

They'd been in Cardiff for a couple of months. Jack and Lucy were starting at their new schools.

The family might be woken by a noise at three o'clock in the morning, and Clare would come downstairs and find Joe stumbling around drunk, looking for money, stashing drugs, vomiting, passing out. Or else sitting in the kitchen with 'the last people you'd want in your house'.

He befriended a teenage boy from a broken home in Caerphilly. 'He was a nice enough kid,' Clare tells me. 'But scary, too. He wore tin foil on his head to keep the rays out of his brain. Joe had replaced his rich-kids-gone-wild friends from the States with people living on the fringes of society.'

He was constantly in trouble with the police for shoplifting, and on one occasion was even picked up for suspiciously loitering and trying to steal a bicycle from the police bike compound. He'd been banned from a number of supermarkets and was currently bailed to appear in Cardiff Youth Court. It wasn't sustainable. Something had to give.

Ed reasoned that Joe rarely stayed at home anyway. He preferred to spend his nights in a squat across town. He also had a girlfriend for a while, who he would sometimes stay with. He'd become gaunt because he wasn't really eating properly but he was still a good-looking boy. Clare recalls that the girl was a couple of years older. She was sweet and seemed fond of him. Then one night Clare got a phone call from her asking if someone could come and pick him up. She still lived with her parents and Joe was too drunk. He'd vomited, couldn't speak. They didn't want him in the house. 'That relationship fizzled out.' Clare's voice cracks a little and she looks away. 'I think she realised that she could probably do better. At least he had a girlfriend in his life.'

Clare is speaking so quietly it's hard to hear her. She reflects on this, as she does on so much else. 'When you really would rather not be saying something you probably drop your voice a little bit. I'm probably suffering from that at the moment. I think if you say it quietly, it's not as true.'

What Clare doesn't want to be true is that they kicked Joe out of the family home. The deal was he'd be allowed in the house only if Clare was there, in order to have a bath or a hot meal, but he couldn't stay unsupervised, and if he wanted to stay overnight it would need to be in the garage. They put a mattress out there, some blankets.

Clare tells me this through long silences. She's struggling not to cry and as her hair falls across her face I register for the first time where little Joe got his tangle of curls. 'It's one of the hardest parts,' she manages. 'I felt very strongly that . . . we had brought him back to this place where he didn't know anyone, didn't have any roots or anything. And he was still a child. So it was . . . it was really our responsibility to help him as much as we could. And not providing him with the basic kind of roof over his head was a failing in keeping him safe.'

Her distress was physical. Aches and pains all over. She began to spend a lot of time in bed. She was drinking. Just getting up to take Jack and Lucy to school, making sure they were washed and had their packed lunches, took everything she had.

Her plan to get a job hadn't materialised. She was too overwhelmed, too racked with guilt about how they were handling everything.

Joe, meanwhile, disappeared to Cambridgeshire for a few days to hang out with his dad's brother. One night, at a bus stop, he approached a lone twenty-four-year-old woman and grabbed her handbag.

She resisted but Joe was too strong. In the struggle she suffered bruising to her arm, some tissue damage. Joe was later spotted by the police, aimlessly roaming the streets. Upon searching him, they discovered a kitchen knife in his bag.

It was his paternal grandmother who got to the police station first and by this time Joe was grinning and laughing strangely to himself. His grandmother asked: 'Did you do it, Joe?' He turned to her, said, 'No,' then gave her a big wink.

Actually mad

Pending trial, Joe was remanded in custody at a Young Offenders Institution near Huntingdon.

Clare travelled to see him, a three-hour drive to a place she'd never heard of, with her thoughts rushing between fury at what he had done ('How dare he mug someone? That poor girl. What sort of monster . .') and fear for his safety. He was vulnerable, still so young. Locked up with criminals who might easily take advantage of him. Beat him up, hurt him. She needed to keep him safe.

She remembers walking along a corridor, with Alsatian sniffer dogs on either side, through complex locked doors. Her hands trembled as she took the bar of chocolate and cup of tea from the machines. Joe sat opposite her. He was talking about how people were looking at him in a funny way. That they were saying one thing and thinking another.

'Why did you do it, Joe? How could you?'

He shrugged. It wasn't a big deal. Then more of the smirking, the bizarre giggling. Clare feels nauseous just thinking about it. One of the guards had commented on it too, that his behaviour seemed disquietingly odd. In Clare's words: 'I realised he was actually mad.'

The prosecution were pushing for a custodial sentence of two years.

The defence solicitor gestured to Joe in the defendant's box and explained to the judge that though it looked like Joe was smirking, there were in fact some mental health issues that his mother was trying to get him help for; help that he obviously needed.

Joe avoided a prison sentence and was ordered to attend a weekly community-based young offenders programme, but over the next few months he continued to deteriorate rapidly. Clare tried and failed to get him the right support. She was in a constant state of anxiety, always waiting for the phone to ring with terrible news. Often she didn't know where Joe was, and at nights would drive around the streets of Cardiff looking for him, showing his photograph at the Salvation Army night bus, where Joe would sometimes go to warm himself up with cups of sugary tea.

'Has anyone seen my son? I'm worried about my son.'

When he did come home – still to be supervised – his memory was poor and he was unable to concentrate, even to play the computer games that he'd so often found refuge and enjoyment in.

He was a couple of months shy of his seventeenth birthday when in the early hours of the morning Clare received a phone call from the local police station. Joe had been arrested for stealing food from a shop. The voice at the other end of the phone explained that Joe was being held in a cell, but that the senior officer on duty had decided he wasn't fit to be interviewed, and that they were arranging for a psychiatrist to come across from the hospital to assess him.

In the official psychiatric report ordered by the Coroner's Court after Joe's death, some details of this early assessment are included:

Mr H— was displaying very incongruent behaviour. He was laughing and giggling inappropriately. He appeared 'void of emotions' in that he was unable to express any concern for himself or anybody else. There appeared to be a delayed response to questioning. It was believed at that time that Mr H— had been using illegal substances and that this was the reason for his presentation. However, a drug screen at the time of the first interview proved negative and he was therefore reassessed and detained under Section 2 of the Mental Health Act on 9th March 2007.

'Have you come to give me some diazies?' Joe asked the nurse who knocked on his bedroom door at the start of the morning shift.

'Are you feeling anxious?' the nurse asked.

'Yeah,' Joe said.

'How does that feel?'

Joe laughed, pressed his face into the pillow. 'I don't know the symptoms.'

His early interactions with the nursing staff on the ward, as recorded in his hospital notes, were almost exclusively limited to him asking for diazepam – an addictive benzodiazepine (commonly known as Valium) that is used to treat anxiety and has a street value for its enjoyable sedative effects.

On one occasion a student nurse tried to engage Joe in a conversation about his life plans. 'Yeah, I've got them,' Joe offered. 'I'm gonna hang around the streets smoking blow.' The student challenged Joe, said that didn't sound like such a good plan. 'Well give me some diazepam then,' Joe replied.

Similar conversations appear daily through his notes, as do observations from the staff that Joe appeared distracted or was smiling and laughing inappropriately, although he did not appear to be responding to visual or auditory hallucinations and did not describe having any unusual beliefs.

Clare and I sit in my car, in the hospital car park, looking up at an ugly, grey building with smeared windows. The inpatient acute psychiatric ward has been closed down for a number of years now – relocated to a newer building in another hospital on the other side of Cardiff – but Clare brings me to see it from the outside. She points up at one of the windows on the second floor. 'Maybe that one was Joe's bedroom. Or the one next to it.'

It was to be his home for the next seven months, as his newly appointed psychiatrist – the one who had assessed him in the police station – tried to figure out what was going on with him, and how to treat it.

Those first weeks Joe spent most of his time pacing the corridors or sitting in the TV room, chain-smoking. He also spent a lot of time dozing or sleeping in his room, sweating into the sheets of his metal-framed bed. There was a small sink in the corner. The bedside table was bolted to the wall.

For Clare, it was a huge relief that Joe was in hospital. She knew where he was. Knew that he was getting help from professionals. Something was being done at last. She even felt strong enough to return to work, accepting a part-time job in research administration. She rediscovered a sense of purpose in her life beyond worrying about Joe and desperately trying to hold her family together.

She would get on the train, look out the window and watch the world slide by.

Everything was going to be sorted. It was all going to be fine.

Hebephrenic schizophrenia

The working diagnosis was arrived at quickly, although due to Joe's young age it was a while before it was made official in his notes. The psychiatric report provided to the Coroner's Court confirms:

> Mr H— fulfilled the criteria for a diagnosis of hebephrenic schizophrenia. This is a disorder that has mainly prominent affective changes showing flattening and incongruity of affect (flattened and sometimes inappropriate emotional response) with behaviour that is often aimless rather than goal directed. There is a tendency towards social isolation and irresponsible behaviour with development of prominent negative symptoms.

Delusions and hallucinations and other positive symptoms of schizophrenia such as auditory hallucinations are usually fleeting.

Mr H—'s mental health was compounded by poly-substance and alcohol misuse.

I wonder how Clare felt that first time she heard the diagnoses mooted? This was during one of the weekly 'ward round' meetings that she attended in order to speak with Joe's consultant psychiatrist.

'You know what,' she tells me. 'That was an *absolutely huge* thing. Ed and I were both able to go from feeling really angry with Joe for behaving so badly, and guilty about ourselves failing as parents, to thinking: Oh! This is why it all happened. He wasn't able to control himself. The illness is what made him do those things.'

An illness, which Clare optimistically assumed would be cured, or at least that the symptoms would be dramatically improved. Then she and Ed did their own reading around it; late-night Google searches, ordering psychiatric journals. The more they read, the more Clare's optimism was chipped away. They discovered that prognosis for hebephrenic schizophrenia was extremely poor. Their expectations were, in Clare's words, 'swiftly managed downwards'. Perhaps Joe would never be a fully independent adult. But surely they could still aim for some semblance of normality, an improvement, at least, on where things were right now.

Side effects

After a while Joe started coming home for weekends.

Clare tells me how he'd changed. She uses words like *drugged* and *aimless* and *lumbering* and *slow*. 'He'd put on weight really quickly,' she tells me. 'He couldn't string two thoughts or words together, really. Yeah, he was . . .' She trails off.

The last flickers of her child disappeared, never to return.

And to what does she attribute that?

Clare doesn't hesitate. 'To the medication,' she says. 'It was the medication.'

A nursing note from early in Joe's admission to hospital reads: '[Joe was] excitable when receiving evening medication. Presume that Joe is not fully informed regarding the nature of his medication and assumed it to be a benzodiazepine.'

Joe was in fact being treated with an antipsychotic medication called risperidone. Over the coming months, he would also be tried on two more, broadly similar medications: quetiapine and olanzapine. The common side effects of these medicines vary, but general themes include anxiety, sleepiness, blurred vision, shaking or tremor, sweating, nausea, dizziness, depression, headache, vomiting, increased saliva production or dry mouth, appetite changes, restlessness, light-headedness, rash, stomach pain or upset, fatigue, trouble sleeping and weight gain.

But did they help?

'Some of them helped a bit,' Clare tells me. 'And there was one that helped quite a lot. I could see his thought processes becoming better, that little spark of intelligence.'

That was the quetiapine, and while Joe was on it Clare recalls that she could sit with him on the ward and talk with him a little about what he was doing in there, what he might want to work towards.

But there were side effects that Joe wouldn't discuss with his mum, and it was Joe who asked that his prescription be changed. His psychiatrist was happy enough for another switch to be made, perhaps because it had been noted that Joe was being increasingly hostile in his attitude to the staff. Clare believes this was because he was becoming more alert to his situation, questioning why he was detained. 'They want compliant patients,' Clare tells me. 'Maybe if we'd had a lot of money and he could go to a private place then those things would have been different. But . . .' Her voice becomes quiet again: 'That wasn't how it worked out.' With the other medications Joe couldn't think beyond the day. His next tablet, his next meal and, increasingly, his next drink.

Under the terms of the Mental Health Act, Joe was forbidden from leaving the ward unescorted but he didn't pay much heed to that. The doors were locked but one way or another he frequently managed to escape. Clare chuckles to herself, with a hint of pride: 'I don't know how.'

He'd escape to get drunk. To find local pubs or parks and drink himself into oblivion. It's been such a theme in his young life and I wonder if Clare has any thoughts on it. What compelled Joe to constantly seek out alcohol and drugs?

She's clear in her own mind, and it's a theory shared by some of the neuroscience papers on the subject, papers that Ed in particular immersed himself in; his own way of coping with what was happening. Something felt wrong in Joe's brain, and had done since his early adolescence. He couldn't articulate it. It may have been at a neurocellular level. Some studies – though there's no consensus on this – point to a critical loss of function in chandelier cells: mysterious, ornately branched interneurons that operate in the cerebral cortex, that part of the brain responsible for higher logic, language, thought, sensation, personality. This loss in function may be counteracted, temporarily at least, with the ingestion of alcohol and nicotine – the two substances that Joe mostly deeply and consistently craved.

'It fulfilled some sort of need in him,' Clare believes. 'Something felt wrong in his head that he wanted to change.'

In other words: Joe was self-medicating.

Three o'clock on a Friday afternoon

He stood outside the ward, clutching a single black bin bag containing everything he owned.

The door was locked behind him.

He was terrified.

It had been a long time coming. Seven months on the acute ward; a further six months on a mental health rehabilitation ward, situated in a normal house, where they aim to get people with chronic mental health problems ready for independent living. 'Teaching basic skills like how to cook a meal, how to live socially, how to sign on, how to go shopping, how to not nick your housemate's milk.' Finally, seven months back on an acute ward, after it became clear that Joe's drinking was spiralling out of control. And after hundreds of cigarette butts were found on his bedroom floor and he was deemed to present a fire hazard.

He'd been tried on a fourth antipsychotic medication. This was clozapine. It was significant because it's used for 'treatment resistant schizophrenia', as the final medication that gets tried if none of the others have worked, but it's recommended not to be mixed with alcohol as this can increase side effects. The nurses on the unit were, as Clare recalls, frightened on Joe's behalf. They were giving him medication that they had serious reservations about; anxious that, given the huge amounts Joe was drinking, the risks to his health were simply too high. Joe's psychiatrist arrived at the same conclusion and the treatment was stopped. In a confidential investigation carried out by the NHS Trust after Joe's death, it was acknowledged that 'There is evidence of confusion in referring to substance misuse services for input.' Joe's mental health issues and alcohol dependence were treated, according to Clare, 'completely separately', though she believes them to have been inextricably linked. That's why she considers that the contract Joe was required to sign during his final weeks in hospital was 'setting him up to fail'. It was a contract whereby he agreed that if he continued to drink he would be discharged.

Many of the nurses on the ward who worked most closely with Joe, who recognised his vulnerability and were fond of him, resisted the decision. This too was acknowledged in the Trust's own confidential investigation:

> The decision to [use a] contract, with discharge being the negative outcome, appears not to have been wholeheartedly supported by all staff. The decision is not documented as having been clearly risk assessed: Mr H— was 19 years of age and had spent the last 18 months as an inpatient with no experience of independent living, had poor daily living skills as assessed in his earlier rehabilitation placement, no clear address (including hostel accommodation) was located and he continued displays of aggressive behaviour on the ward. No alternative care plan was identified for any precipitated discharge.
>
> The decision to discharge on a Friday afternoon left no time to put in place any support immediately post discharge.

There was no plan in place for him beyond a taxi being called to take him to a homeless shelter. Joe was convinced he would be beaten up the moment he arrived. No way was he going there. He'd rather sleep under a bush.

'They'd given up on him,' Clare tells me. 'And part of the reason I think was because they were under a lot of pressure for bed space. They decided he wasn't worth spending their resources on. I was furious and scared. And powerless; there's nothing you can do. What the fuck are we going to do?'

All my love, Mum

The last time Clare saw her son alive, they went for lunch together in a cafe. That's what Joe wanted to do. It was a summer afternoon. There were chairs outside, and Clare felt relieved that they wouldn't need to go indoors.

Joe never used the bath in the small private flat she had secured for him after he was kicked off the ward ten long months before. She'd had to lie to get him that flat. She'd said he was a student, but was currently ill and was taking a term out. There were no other options. Ed still wouldn't let Joe live at home. The waiting lists for specialist supported housing were *years* long. Once a week, Clare took Joe along to the outpatient mental health team, where she would openly weep in meetings. She wept as the doctor explained the results of Joe's latest liver function test. His lifestyle was having a devastating effect on his physical health. The doctor started to talk about a shortened life expectancy. She spoke about the next three to five years.

'Nobody asked if I would like to go and talk to somebody,' Clare tells me. 'Not a single person said, "Oh, you know what? You could really do with some help, too."' These months were characterised for her by a profound sense of loneliness, but it never occurred to her to seek help for herself. *It's worse for Joe.* That's all she could think. *It's worse for Joe. It's worse for Joe.*

She looked across the cafe table at him, at the food smeared down his top and stuck in his beard. He was fidgeting, had a noticeable tremor in his hand. His breathing was shallow. He looked like he was struggling not to have a panic attack.

It was scary for Joe to leave his flat; to step outside into a world where he was increasingly certain people wanted to hurt him.

He'd stopped opening his door to the community mental health nurse who visited once a week, knocked a few times, then left.

'I'm drinking because my life's so shit,' Joe told his mum, staring blankly ahead. 'It's the only good thing in my life.'

They talked on the phone a couple of days later. Joe wanted a fiver so he could buy some bottles of cider.

Clare didn't have time for this, not right now. There were other things going on. Ed was having issues at work, which they were locked into a heated argument over. It was the summer holidays. Lucy and Jack needed attention, too. Joe would have to wait.

She called him later that day but he didn't answer. He didn't answer the next day either. She and Ed knocked on the door of his flat. They called through the letterbox, could hear the radio playing inside.

He was still mates with the young lad from Caerphilly, the one who wore the tin foil on his head. He and Joe took a lot of drugs together.

Bloody Joe, Clare told herself. *Off up to no good again*. But she couldn't convince herself, or ignore the undercurrent of worry.

They left a bag of sandwiches hanging on his door handle, and turned away.

It was the landlord who unlocked the door in the end. Ed unscrewed the security chain. Clare stayed at home with Jack and Lucy.

She phoned Ed for the third time, and once again rang through to answerphone.

She knew. She'd known all along.

Today, I meet with Clare at her home. She has recently moved house following her separation from Ed and there are still some things in boxes. She digs out a heavy cardboard box, bulging with paperwork. The lid won't close properly.

She can't bring herself to look through it, but neither does she want to throw it out. She decides that handing it over to me to help with my research feels like a good way of letting it go.

We're interrupted when Lucy trundles down the stairs and chats with us briefly. She's sixteen, waiting for her GCSE results. She's expected to ace them. She takes after her mum. In the corner of the room is a piano, and her Grade Six certificate.

After Lucy leaves us, Clare tells me how a couple of weeks ago she came down for breakfast wearing a pair of sweatpants that looked immediately familiar. Clare held her breath. She had no idea they still existed, that they'd been kept this whole time. They never fitted Joe properly. He bought them off another patient on one of the wards for way too much money.

Clare told Lucy that they once belonged to her big brother. She's carried on wearing them. Joe's never that far away.

The box is mostly filled with the reams of hospital notes, medication charts, police reports, bail applications, care plans and various other documents that followed Joe through the final years of his life, along with the official inquests and correspondence that sought to make sense of his death.

There are other things, too, including things that Clare hadn't realised were in there. There are more photographs of Joe, a certificate he was awarded upon graduating from middle school and some positive school reports from when he was little, including one from a Grade Three teacher expressing how much she enjoyed teaching 'Joey'.

I tell Clare about these and on a subsequent visit we go through the box together to remove them. She wants to put them in another box that she's keeping. This one is smaller and much less full. 'He had so few possessions in the end,' she tells me. 'Nothing really salvageable, the flat was such a mess.'

She's kept his fake Zippo lighter, complete with cannabis leaf embossed on the side. His tobacco tin, wallet, mobile phone. There's a small trophy that he won with a youth basketball team as a little boy. There's some dried foliage taken from the wreath at his funeral.

With the new things added the box appears fuller. 'That looks better, doesn't it?' Clare asks.

It does. And I feel both utterly heartbroken and profoundly privileged to share in this moment.

Also in that box is a letter to Joe, written by Clare:[1]

You are always hovering in the background of my thoughts as I wake in the morning and go to sleep at night, but I'm writing this now as I realise that your 21st birthday is coming up and I don't know what I'm going to do on that day.

Since that awful moment we found you dead nearly 18 months ago, I have realised I had been grieving for the handsome, happy and exuberant boy that I lost to mental illness for much longer. I know you'll agree that your teenage years were hard on us all, most especially you, but you never recognised the devastating extent of the heartache you caused me. On that day the worst happened, I was able to stop worrying about what would happen to you, and among the terrible pain and sadness there was also relief. After all, it could have been much worse, and had been many times in my imagination. Once, you said that if I chose to worry it was my problem, not yours. Your selfishness greatly frustrated me.

You didn't often realise anything was wrong with your life, but it was hard to be close to you and watch the rapid deterioration in your personality, and intellect, and the complete lack of purpose and ambition left within you.

My aspirations for you dwindled until my only aim was that you were reasonably content and did no harm. You were so big (whatever they say, your massive weight increase was caused by the antipsychotic medication you depended on) and difficult to love unconditionally near the end, that I failed to realise – or wouldn't admit – just how vulnerable you were.

So the main reason I wanted to write was to say sorry. I did the best I could with you and for you at the time, but it wasn't good enough and I ultimately failed to protect you and keep you safe. I wish I could go back in time and do things differently.

I also wanted to ask you about what happened at the end. It's still not clear, despite an inquest. It seems as if you fell and banged your head, and then your heart just gave up, your body weakened by alcohol and the medication you took faithfully, and which I now wish you hadn't. I hope with all my heart that you slipped away quietly and with some clarity and relief. I'm both glad your life as it was has ended and for ever full of sorrow that you are gone.

All my love, Mum

Causes

IT'S HARD TO KNOW WHAT TO SAY, ISN'T IT? That's what we're dealing with here. Broken young men dropping dead in their flats. Joe is not a statistic. At the same time, his story does not exist in isolation.

Someone living today in the UK with a diagnosis of schizophrenia has a life expectancy that's twenty years shorter than that of the general population.[1]

In the context of what happened to Joe, and the grief that Clare must navigate every single day of her life, my earlier discussions about diagnostic labelling feel almost absurd in their abstraction.

In fact, Joe's diagnosis illustrates this perfectly. Since his death, 'hebephrenic schizophrenia' has technically ceased to exist. It never made the cut for DSM-5. Along with the other so-called subtypes of schizophrenia, including 'paranoid schizophrenia', it has now been consigned to history. Those most critical of psychiatric diagnostics may see this as a victory – evidence that such terms were meaningless, as they will all ultimately prove to be – whereas those who seek to defend diagnostics may see it as evidence that we are continuing to both expand and refine our understanding; such subtypes, it was argued, did not adequately reflect the heterogeneity of the disorder, nor meaningfully predict its course or inform its treatment.[2] Better to drop them and to focus our attention on the *real* schizophrenia.

Truths change over time. Meanwhile, Joe remains dead. And Clare continues to live with that concrete, absolute and unalterable fact.

So I will now respectfully turn our attention away from the ongoing debates over what labels, if any, we should ascribe to this particular kind of suffering, and begin to consider instead the question of what causes it. What causes people to fall apart in this way: to disconnect from their friends, their families and their reality? What causes people to retreat into themselves, sometimes never to return?

To try to answer this we need first to set our parameters. As we've learnt from the stories we've heard so far, the suffering endured by people with so-called schizophrenia can extend far beyond the direct effects of what might be considered its core symptoms. The hard reality of discrimination, for instance, may well prove more intolerable to someone than the demonstrable falsehood of their delusions. And failings in our health services, stemming from their own myriad of complex causes, might result in greater distress and confusion for a person than the cruel words uttered by any voices in their head. It is also possible, as we will discover later in this book, that some of the distressing experiences that we might think of as being absolutely intrinsic to 'schizophrenia' are the result not of some underlying disorder, but rather of the very medicines that are intended to treat it.

Accepting, then, that the catalysts for this kind of suffering don't all arrive in a single moment, we still need to start our enquiry somewhere.

I find myself thinking of Joe again.

'Joey', his Grade Three teacher called him. A happy, energetic and exuberant little boy. And the honest truth is that my mind drifts to my own two happy, energetic and exuberant little children. Something changed somewhere for Joe and that frightens me. Was it always lurking in the shadows? Was his script written from the start?

The circumstances and events of Joe's short life – along with the other stories we've heard – point us towards a few of the main causal theories of so-called schizophrenia and 'mental illness' more generally. A crucial thing to remember, though, is that they are just that: *theories*.

Also, what the science can tell us is currently only applicable at a 'population level'. This means that we've identified a number of *trends* by looking at large numbers of people but we are not yet in a position where we can confidently apply these trends to *individuals*.

As things stand, no mental health professional, of any persuasion, can say to an *individual* patient (or service user or survivor or journalist or soldier or son) that they *know* what caused them to develop 'schizophrenia' or, for that matter, 'depression', 'anxiety', 'obsessive–compulsive disorder' and so on. That's a simple truth which sometimes gets lost in what are often emotive and highly charged conversations, both for mental health professionals and for people who live with a mental illness diagnosis.*

Before setting out to write this essay, I met with Clare and together we listed some of the main causal theories of 'mental illness' as she understood them. Clare talked about genetics and the fact that Joe's biological father had a schizophrenia diagnosis. We discussed neurological theories, as hypothesised by Joe's stepdad, and the risks associated with certain recreational drugs.

I'll explore each of these in a moment. First, I want to reflect upon where our conversation went next.

I wanted to speak with Clare about another theory, which is that

---

* This seems as good a time as any to state the obvious fact that being a mental health professional and suffering from poor mental health are not mutually exclusive positions. That's another simple truth that often gets lost, to the detriment of all concerned.

adverse life events during childhood – and any trauma associated with these – are widely considered to increase our risk of experiencing all kinds of mental health problems.[3] In fact, not just mental health problems. Childhood adversity, including being subject to abuse and living in an environment with sustained exposure to parental conflicts, plays a role in cancer, respiratory disease, heart disease, problematic drug and alcohol misuse use and violence.[4] In this respect, it's my opinion that cruelty to children is not just abominable in and of itself, it's also a major public health issue.

Too many young children endure horrific upbringings, and we know that physical, sexual and emotional abuse, neglect and bullying substantially increase the risk of the child growing up to suffer from psychosis.[5] Child sex abuse, in particular, has been shown to strongly correlate with devastatingly poorer mental health outcomes.* As a nation, we are only beginning to wake up to the sheer scale of this. The NSPCC estimates that one in twenty children in the UK have been sexually abused,[6] and one review found that between half and three quarters of psychiatric inpatients had suffered sexual or physical abuse as children.[7]

You know what, I'm going to say that again:

---

* The reason that we talk about *correlation* rather than concluding that child abuse is an independent *cause* of 'mental illness' is because it's often impossible for researchers to disentangle any potential effects of abuse from the potential effects of confounding variables. For example, people who describe having been the victims of childhood sexual abuse also frequently – though, of course, not always – describe having been raised in disadvantaged or broken homes where a whole range of dysfunctional family dynamics, conflicts and poor parenting practices are thrown into the mix. So we cannot say with complete certainty that it was sexual abuse that caused, say, psychosis or anxiety, over and above some other factor or combination of factors. These are the limitations of this kind of science. However, from a personal perspective I believe the best approach is to simply ask people what they believe is causing them to feel the way they do, listen without prejudice, and move forwards from there.

The NSPCC estimates that one in twenty children in the UK have been sexually abused, and one review found that between half and three quarters of psychiatric inpatients had suffered sexual or physical abuse as children.

However shocking these figures, for many of us it will still make intuitive sense that such brutal childhood trauma leaves deep and lasting wounds, even if we do not fully understand – as nobody does – the specific biological pathways that turn this trauma into the symptoms of a given mental disorder.

What may be more difficult to comprehend, though, are the far-reaching consequences of childhood experiences that do not, on the face of it, appear to be so intensely traumatic. Something as commonplace as separation from a parent, for instance, increases our vulnerability to even the most serious mental health problems, with some research suggesting that people who experience a psychotic episode are around 2.4 times more likely to have been separated from one or both parents by the age of sixteen.[*8] It was this general discussion that I'd hoped to have with Clare, rather than any specific dissection of Joe's childhood. Yet I found myself feeling unusually hesitant, unable to think of the right words.

In truth, I was afraid that to raise even the smallest possibility that events in Joe's life may have contributed to him becoming unwell might be interpreted by Clare as me seeking to point the finger of blame.

---

* It's important for us to remember that even if a person is two or three times more likely than the general population to develop so-called schizophrenia, the odds are still highly favourable that they won't. As a ballpark figure, one in every hundred people receives the diagnosis. Treble the risk and we're looking at a three-in-a-hundred chance.

Not so long ago, mental health professionals had strong form when it came to the practice of blaming parents – and especially mothers – for causing their children to develop schizophrenia. This was the prevailing orthodoxy (most notably in the United States) during psychiatry's love affair with psychoanalysis between the late 1940s and 1970s.

It was during this time that the ugly concept of the 'schizo-phrenogenic mother' emerged. Mothers could get nothing right. They either drove their children mad by not caring enough, or else they were too caring. Either way, in some bafflingly Freudian and transparently misogynistic sense it was *all their fault*. The aca-demic neuropsychologist Simon McCarthy-Jones argues that such unsubstantiated claims caused an entirely justified backlash that contributed to the ideological pendulum swinging far in the oppo-site direction. In the US, families formed powerful lobbying groups which unsurprisingly rejected the notion that parents could have a role in causing mental illness, gravitating instead to the emerging biological explanations. Such campaign groups received significant donor funding from the pharmaceutical industry, which for obvious reasons was also keen on champion-ing this message. We've already talked about the similarly shifting position of psychiatry with the publication of DSM-III, and so, as McCarthy-Jones explains, parents and psychiatry now partnered against the finger-pointing, mother-shaming narrative of psycho-analysis, giving the biomedical model of schizophrenia 'a potent mix of political, moral and scientific authority'.[9]

Perhaps the pendulum is now slowly – too slowly for many – swinging back to its centre, especially in the UK, where in recent years there's been a move within some NHS Mental Health Trusts towards what's broadly termed 'trauma-informed practice'.[10] Part of this approach involves mental health nurses and other professionals receiving better training in how to explore issues of child abuse and neglect.

Hold up! you might be thinking. *Surely, addressing traumatic childhoods is already the mainstay of therapeutic chit-chats up and down the country.* You'd be forgiven for assuming this but it's not the case. Most people who use mental health services are never asked about child abuse or neglect, and men diagnosed with psychotic disorders (including schizophrenia) are the least likely to be asked.[11]

In my own experience of nursing in acute psychiatric settings, I never felt especially confident about how to approach or handle such conversations, and there was a general sense on the wards that our patients were simply too disturbed, too psychotic or too afraid to meaningfully address traumatic memories which, in the short term, might only compound their distress.

It may also be psychiatry's shameful hangover from having invented the schizophrenogenic mother that has left some professionals with the belief that certain subjects are simply taboo. As Anne Harrington writes in the *Lancet*: 'Fear of giving any energy to discredited models of family blaming means that, today, cultural and psychosocial questions relating to schizophrenia are rarely discussed.'[12]

All the more reason to discuss them now.

A bit more cultural and psychosocial stuff

The single strongest predictor of psychosis and so-called schizophrenia, according to Professor of Clinical Psychology John Read, is poverty. This is not because poverty in itself is a cause of any of these outcomes, but rather because it is, he suggests, *the cause of causes*.

Living in poverty increases a person's likely exposure to a whole range of stressors and potentially traumatising events, while simultaneously reducing access to resources that might help us overcome these.

In fact, the only predictor that Read deems to be stronger than *absolute poverty* is *relative poverty*. Wealthy nations with the greatest income inequality have the highest prevalence of so-called mental illness, with rates that are around five times higher in the most unequal compared to the least unequal societies. Unsurprisingly, Britain and the US are among the world's most unequal and most mentally unwell nations.

We do not fully understand the pathways by which inequality exerts its effects, though as social creatures human beings seem hard-wired to be conscious of our status in relation to others – and so it's suggested that our mental health suffers greatly when poverty excludes us from community life and a sense of being socially valued.[13]

Though those on the bottom rungs of the economic ladder undoubtedly suffer most cruelly, inequality is a source of mental stress and anguish for everyone living in unequal societies, regardless of their personal living standards.[14] There are no winners where we allow for there to be losers.

It's a disturbing fact that there are higher rates of diagnosed psychotic disorders among minority ethnic groups, and in the UK this is especially so for second-generation African Caribbeans. This has led many to conclude that psychiatry is institutionally racist, and to accuse psychiatrists of viewing culturally unfamiliar expressions of distress through the narrow lens of Western values and assumptions.

There's something important to tease apart here, because although institutional racism may lead to heavy-handed diagnostics and treatment (and I believe it does result in these things, which we'll revisit later) that does not in itself explain why more young black men – especially those living in urban environments – have the kind of strange experiences that place them in front of psychiatrists and mental health teams in the first place.

What might better explain this, according to Dr Lucy Johnstone and colleagues, is that these young men are often living at the point where multiple forms of disadvantage and discrimination intersect.[15]

This isn't – to borrow a phrase from Professor of Social and Community Psychiatry Swaran Singh – 'a black-and-white issue'. He notes that rates of psychotic disorders are disproportionately high not just among the African-Caribbean community in the UK, but for all immigrant groups globally.

Some of the highest reported rates of psychosis are among Greenlanders in Denmark. Rates are also high among Finnish migrants to Sweden, and in British, German, Polish and Italian migrants in Australia. The issue, Professor Singh suggests, is one of social discrimination and adversity. Migrant groups are more likely to face repeated experiences of marginalisation and exclusion leading to what he calls 'social defeat'. There is even evidence that staying in the same country but moving home or schools several times during adolescence increases the risk of psychosis. As Singh explains: 'Every time you move schools you leave your peer group and your support network, and you start again as an outsider. So it's that chronic experience of being an outsider which we think is related to the development of psychosis.'[16]

Even if we don't move around, where we live still influences our mental wellbeing. On the whole, urban living doesn't seem especially good for the human mind.

Men living in the most densely populated regions of Sweden, for example, are at a 68 per cent higher risk of becoming psychotic than those living in the countryside. For women the risk is 77 per cent higher. Both sexes are also markedly more likely to be depressed.[17] And a recent study examining incidence of treated psychosis across seventeen sites in six countries revealed that someone living in South London is eight times more likely to become psychotic than someone living in Santiago in Spain. Such huge variations remain even after researchers take race and ethnicity out of the equation.[18]

'That can't be genetic,' says Professor Robin Murray, who was one of the study's authors. 'It's very unlikely it's genetic. It's probably social fragmentation and the effect of the inner city. And it's probably cannabis. So we ought to be able to do something about that.'

Ah, yes. Cannabis.

It's all but obligatory for liberal folk (and I count myself as one) to speak out in favour of cannabis being less damaging than alcohol. For society as a whole it absolutely is less damaging, but that doesn't mean it's not deeply problematic for some people – and possibly for more people than we'd like to imagine.

Between 2005 and 2011, patients at the Maudsley psychiatric hospital in South London were asked about whether they smoked cannabis, the frequency of their use, and what type of cannabis they used. The results showed a strong correlation between becoming psychotic and smoking cannabis every day. Curiously, though, this was only the case for people who smoked the high-potency form of cannabis, known as skunk. People who smoked the more natural strain of cannabis, known as hash, were no more likely to become psychotic than people who didn't use cannabis at all.[19]

The main psychoactive ingredient in skunk – which may also be the main ingredient involved in inducing psychosis – is tetra-hydrocannabinol (THC). Skunk is high in THC content, at the expense of other naturally occurring molecules. One of these natural molecules found in hash is cannabidiol (CBD), which remarkably appears to protect against the harmful psychosis-inducing effects of THC.*[20]

This discovery has led to ongoing research into whether CBD could be used as an antipsychotic medication in its own right. Either way, it appears to be unbalanced products such as skunk – which contain only traces of CBD and are high in THC – that present the greatest risk to mental health.[21] Indeed, the researchers at the Maudsley estimate that 24 per cent of cases of first-presentation psychosis could be prevented if skunk were removed from the equation.

As ever, though, things aren't quite so clear-cut as they first appear. As we've seen with the tragic example of child abuse, proving a correlation is not the same as proving causation. 'For all sorts of reasons, you can't randomly assign one group of teenagers to use cannabis, and another not to,' explains Dr Suzi Gage, presenter of the award-winning podcast *Say Why to Drugs*. 'This means you have to observe what people choose to do, and the people who choose to smoke cannabis might be different in a variety of other ways, which could be the cause of the increase in psychosis risk.' Also, she points out, this study didn't test cannabis samples, it only asked people to remember what kind of cannabis they used to smoke in the past, which they might not always recall accurately. Notwithstanding that, she writes, 'Just

---

* This is proof, if ever it were needed, that Mother Nature is a sweetheart and that we should stop dumping plastic in her oceans.

in the same way that a pint of beer of an evening is likely to have a different health impact to a pint of vodka, the same could be true for skunk compared to hash.'[22]

This all leads me to wonder whether for some people environmental factors alone – our childhoods, where we live, how much money we have, what drugs we take – could be enough to cause so-called schizophrenia without us needing to have any biological predisposition whatsoever?

It's a question I pose to Professor Robin Murray. He's cautious but doesn't rule it out.

He suggests that for some of his patients, growing up in Lambeth in South London may itself be enough to lead towards psychosis. 'You're brought up maybe in a one-parent family,' he says. 'You have lousy schooling, you have lousy housing, you don't get educated. You leave school early. You don't get a job. If you're black, the police pick you up. I don't know whether if you had absolutely no genetic susceptibility you would still tip into psychosis. But I think these are the sort of questions we'll have the answer to in five years.'

That's encouraging, though having spoken with many, many health scientists, I should possibly add that 'five years' does seem to be the standard unit of time after which *all things will be known*. There's also the well-documented 'seventeen-year lag', which is widely considered to be the average length of time it takes for health professionals to change their practice after a new scientific discovery is made.

Take all this to its logical conclusion and in twenty-two years' time we'll have understood and cured all human morbidity.

Shall we hold our breath?

And now some biological stuff

Mercifully, most people who suffer even the most horrendous life events such as child abuse do not go on to develop the so-called serious mental disorders. Neither do most people who have been bullied, displaced, brought up in poverty or smoke cannabis every day.

Those people who do become unwell will not inevitably experience the same disorders or suffer them to the same degree. And although if we expand the definition of 'trauma' far enough then we will inevitably all have experienced it in some form or other, it would be a stretch, and a stretch into the absurd, to conclude that trauma and environmental pressures are the only relevant causal factors for *every* individual.

Most likely there's an important interaction at play between our environment and our genes. Following my conversations with Clare, I arranged to meet with the psychiatric geneticist Professor James Walters. As it happens, I didn't need to travel too far. The MRC Centre for Neuropsychiatric Genetics and Genomics is the largest psychiatric genetics group in the UK, and is situated in Cardiff.

Professor Walters is Cardiff born and bred. His nan, he tells me, was a cook at Whitchurch Hospital, one of the hospitals (and, it should be added, one of the better ones according to Clare) in which Joe received his treatment. From when he was very young, James Walters was taken along to collect his nan from work every Sunday. It was a ritual that went on for years. He remembers hanging out with the patients and staff. He was fascinated by the place. He can't now recall a time when he didn't want to be a psychiatrist.

Much like the other experts we've so far encountered, Professor Walters does not consider schizophrenia to be a discrete pathological entity and neither is he a great fan of the categorical system of diagnosis, particularly for the genetic research that he conducts. He introduces me to the idea of a 'dimensional approach': instead of grouping together the *presence* or *absence* of so-called symptoms (such as low mood and paranoid thoughts) and putting these into potentially arbitrary boxes with names like 'bipolar' and 'schizophrenia', we could concentrate on the *degree* to which said symptoms are experienced – as measured on continuums – and not bother with the packaging at all. To this end, I wonder if he agrees with the theory we've heard elsewhere that what we call schizophrenia is in fact nothing more than the severe end of a psychosis spectrum?

'It's not as simple as that,' he suggests. 'Psychosis per se doesn't capture all that we're talking about. It's psychosis *plus* other things. And the most disabling are often the cognitive and negative symptoms.'*

It rings true with what we learnt about Joe. His cognitive decline was devastating. Clare once told me how scary it was the day he forgot how to form the letter R.

After the human genome – the complete set of human DNA – was mapped at the turn of the millennium, there were initial hopes among some genetic scientists that a single faulty gene might be discovered for 'schizophrenia', in the same way as happened for the genetically inherited Huntington's disease – which, incidentally, also has psychosis as one of its many cruel symptoms.

This wasn't an unreasonable hope. The most reliable predictor of developing so-called schizophrenia is having a first-degree relative with it. It runs in families. If you have a biological parent

---

* You will recall that 'negative symptoms' include social withdrawal and a lack of motivation to accomplish even pleasurable tasks.

with a diagnosis of schizophrenia then your odds of landing the same diagnosis are much increased – up to about a thirteen-in-a-hundred chance. However, most people with so-called schizophrenia have no such parent or relative, and in this sense it does not have the same inheritance pattern as simpler genetic conditions like Huntingdon's. Even identical twins show only a slightly higher than 50 per cent concordance rate, meaning that being genetically identical to someone with the disorder still far from guarantees a shared outcome.

We now know there's no single 'schizophrenia gene'. But genes are still important. Recent international studies looking at many tens of thousands of people with 'schizophrenia' have identified more than a hundred genetic variants (or common mutations) spread across the genome that are associated with the disorder. That is to say, they show up significantly more often in people with the diagnosis than people without it. One of the largest and perhaps most groundbreaking of these studies – known as Genome Wide Association Studies – was published in the journal *Nature* in 2014.[23] It was conducted by more than three hundred scientists from thirty-five countries and compared common genetic variants across the whole genomes of nearly thirty-seven thousand people with 'schizophrenia' with those of more than 113,000 controls.* These studies rarely pinpoint specific genes but they have identified *regions* of the genome that we can now be confident are implicated in an increased risk of a person developing 'schizophrenia'.

Some of these identified regions add weight to existing biological

---

* Like all research, genetics research is not without its limitations and it is by no means immune to the trend of declaring major breakthroughs that turn out to be not quite so major as first suggested. To its very real credit, though, it does not mess about with small sample sizes and in this respect is arguably more robust than many other fields of mental health research.

theories. For instance, a longstanding theory (which we'll return to later in this book) is that psychosis is linked to overactive dopamine signalling in the brain. And the Genome Wide Association Studies have indeed implicated regions of the genome containing a gene which produces the exact dopamine receptors thought to be involved in this.

It has also become increasingly clear over the past decade that many of the genes that increase our susceptibility to so-called schizophrenia are also associated with a whole range of other mental health disorders. Chief among these is 'bipolar disorder'. A Swedish population study that examined data from two million families found evidence of a substantial genetic relationship between these two diagnoses, and demonstrated that the children of someone with 'schizophrenia' are at an increased risk of developing either condition.[24] Such family-based studies have recently been supported by molecular genetic research that demonstrates a large overlap between the specific genetic risk variants for 'schizophrenia' and 'bipolar disorder'.[25] Again, this underlines the point that it's almost certainly inaccurate to regard any of these so-called major mental health disorders as standalone diseases.

Professor Walters believes that some of the most interesting and productive work in the field of genetics is the study of copy number variation (CNV). Each of us has a blueprint of about twenty thousand genes and it used to be believed that these genes were almost always present in two copies in a person's genome. We now know this isn't the case. Genes that were thought to always occur in two copies have sometimes been found to be present in one, three or more than three copies. This can be observed in the one in four thousand of us who have 22q11 deletion syndrome. People with this syndrome are missing a part of one copy of chromosome 22 in each cell, containing about thirty to sixty genes. This deletion is strongly correlated with a schizophrenia diagnosis. 'These people have a very high risk of developing psychosis,' James Walters explains. 'About one in three people with 22q11 deletion will develop psychosis. And about one in four will develop schizophrenia.' This has clinical implications. If we know from genetic testing that an individual has such an increased risk of becoming unwell then – theoretically at least – measures can be taken to ensure appropriate support is in place. Curiously enough, people who have 22q11 duplications (i.e. they carry an extra copy of these genes) seem to be protected against developing 'schizophrenia'. This is not without cost, though, and those carrying the duplication are at an increased risk of suffering intellectual disability and autism.[26]

Of course, the fact that a high percentage of people with 22q11 deletion develop so-called schizophrenia does not mean that a high percentage of people with so-called schizophrenia have 22q11 deletion.

'This still only accounts for about 0.3 per cent of the total number of people with schizophrenia,' Professor Walters notes. 'And altogether these rare copy number variants are seen in around 3 per cent of cases. Although there's strong evidence that some CNVs increase the risk of schizophrenia, they also increase the risk of ADHD, autism, intellectual disability and epilepsy. And some people who carry these rare genetic variants seemingly have very few problems. What takes a person in one direction or another will be partly common genetics and partly environmental factors. We cannot talk about genes as being deterministic for such complex conditions. It's just another risk factor or protective factor. Genetics is a small part of a much bigger picture.'

Before we conclude our conversation, James Walters shows me a video that brings a genuine tear to my eye (which I quickly wipe away before it compromises my status as alpha male). The video is a news clip about a summer camp in the US for children diagnosed with Williams Syndrome. These children have a deletion of around twenty-five genes in chromosome 7. The result is that they are almost impossibly friendly towards everyone they meet, as well as extremely curious about them and empathetic. They show unusually enhanced emotional engagement and expressive language. That's what the genetic deletion does, whereas a duplication in the same region is known to be associated with autism and language delay. Professor Walters wants to share this, in part because it shows some of the power of these reciprocal genetic variations in helping us to make sense of the associated features, but also because, as he explains, 'It shows why we need to be very careful in considering genetic variation as only deleterious.'

That's not to say that people with Williams Syndrome are not in any way disadvantaged by their condition. It's still fundamentally a syndrome of learning disability. And it occurred to me immediately upon watching the video that their unusually trusting and friendly disposition would make these children extremely vulnerable to abuse. Though that speaks of a problem with society, not with them, doesn't it?[27]

In the German-occupied Netherlands towards the end of the Second World War, food supplies became dangerously scarce. Accounts from the time reveal that many Dutch people – living on meagre rations of bread and potatoes – were forced to walk tens of kilometres each day in the hope of exchanging their possessions for food. People ate their pets in order to survive. Twenty thousand people died of starvation in what became known as the *Hongerwinter* (literal translation: Hunger Winter).

It was later observed that there were unusually high rates of so-called schizophrenia among people who were conceived during this famine. The same was observed after the Chinese famine of 1959–61.[28] Such is the backdrop for the neurodevelopmental hypothesis of schizophrenia, which posits that – in the case of these famines – undernutrition in the womb could have disturbed foetal brain development, and that a substantial number of people who receive a diagnosis of schizophrenia in adulthood may have suffered some form or other of foetal or early-life brain insult.[29]

Maternal illness during pregnancy (including flu and various viral and bacterial infections) and complications such as pre-eclampsia, premature birth, low birth weight and infant hypoxia have all been implicated in increasing the odds of someone later receiving a schizophrenia diagnosis. So too have certain genes that are known to play an important role in healthy neural functioning, including the migration of new cells within the developing infant brain and the formation of synapses.

These neurodevelopmental theories are perhaps given extra clout by the fact that when we look back through the histories of people with a schizophrenia diagnosis there's often (though certainly not always) evidence of developmental delay in childhood, such as reaching educational milestones later than their peers or not interacting as well socially. Similarly, children who go on to develop 'schizophrenia' often experience a minor drop in IQ compared to their peers years beforehand, all of which suggests that their brains may not have developed in such an efficient way.

The assumption here is that these subtle brain abnormalities caused at the start of life only go on to trigger the symptoms of so-called schizophrenia through a later interaction with the brain's normal maturation process. This may occur during 'synaptic pruning', when our adolescent brain does away with the excess of unused synaptic connections that we form as infants. It may be that unhealthy brains are overly zealous in their pruning, and it's this that causes the array of strange thoughts, feelings and behaviours we call schizophrenia. This could also explain why these symptoms are seldom seen prior to adolescence.[30]

Though such theories have gained traction over recent decades, they're not without their detractors.

'What use is a brain that doesn't react to its environment?' asks John Read, Professor of Clinical Psychology, whom we heard from earlier.

It's his conviction that observed abnormalities in the brain associated with 'schizophrenia' are identical to those effected on the developing brain by early childhood trauma and abuse. He therefore proposes a 'traumagenic neurodevelopmental model', asserting that any brain abnormalities seen in so-called schizophrenia are not necessarily causal and certainly not evidence of brain disease.[31]

We've arrived, it seems, at a chicken-and-egg argument.

And it's a lot to take in, isn't it?

If it's any comfort, when I started this book I had no idea that I was going to get to page 147 and find myself writing the words 'traumagenic neurodevelopmental model'. We don't see that sort of thing coming, do we? It's taken me by surprise.

So if your own brain is swimming a bit then I promise you're not alone. It may also reassure you to know that not everyone working in mental health is preoccupied with the search for causes.

There is a different way of thinking.

A different way of thinking

'I think the search for causes is misguided,' says Dr Joanna Moncrieff.

Since her days at medical school, Dr Moncrieff has always found the mainstream views of psychiatry to be problematic. She recalls her first student placements on psychiatric wards, and how even then it felt clear to her that people were being repressed and restrained rather than treated.

This was in the late 1980s. She was reading the works of Thomas Szasz, a psychiatrist and academic who rejected traditional notions of 'mental illness'. She knew there were different ways of thinking, though at the time she felt she had no choice but to keep her head down and try to pass her exams. Today, she's a consultant psychiatrist and a founding member of the Critical Psychiatry Network, which seeks to challenge the medicalised view of distress.

'I think we should see schizophrenia as a variant of character or personality,' she tells me. 'We could think of it in the same way as other personality traits, such as a tendency to lose one's temper, or being a very impatient person. All of these things may have some biological component and they're going to be influenced by life events. But we're never going to be able to say that this aspect of behaviour is caused by *this* or *this* or *this*. I think it's the same with schizophrenia. Ultimately, it's just a rather mysterious way of being human.'[32]

I like that sentiment, and am reminded of my conversations with the psychologist Dr Lucy Johnstone. We'd talked about how people with a diagnosis of schizophrenia are often very sensitive, picking up on interpersonal vibes and feeling things deeply. To her mind, the mistake geneticists too often make is to conceptualise this as a biological vulnerability to illness rather than a temperamental factor, which in the right circumstances could be a real advantage. We might hope that mental health workers are very sensitive people, for instance, but we do not talk about 'a genetic vulnerability to training as a psychiatric nurse'. In this respect, how we understand a quality such as 'sensitivity' seems mostly to depend on how it plays itself out – and this may be more a reflection of a person's circumstances than it is indicative of anything fundamentally lacking, wrong or deficient about them.

One reason that Joanna Moncrieff is so sceptical about the scientific search for the causes of mental illness is that so far they've made virtually no difference to clinical outcomes. After stepping down from his role as Director of the US National Institute of Mental Health, Thomas Insel conceded:

> I spent 13 years at NIMH really pushing on the neuroscience and genetics of mental disorders, and when I look back on that I realize that while I think I succeeded at getting lots of really cool papers published by cool scientists at fairly large costs — I think $20 billion — I don't think we moved the needle in reducing suicide, reducing hospitalizations, improving recovery for the tens of millions of people who have mental illness.[33]

'I think we need to stop chasing the causes and ask ourselves how do we live with this problem?' says Moncrieff. 'How do we enable people to lead as fulfilling lives as possible? How do we identify what makes it difficult for people with these particular characteristics to function in our society? And might there be ways of organising society that would make it easier for them?'

They're questions worth thinking about because right now our society doesn't seem well organised on that front at all.

As we'll now confront, all too often, our society turns its back.

THE COMMUNITY

Moving statues

IN THE SUMMER OF 1985 in the Irish village of Ballinspittle, County Cork, two teenage girls reported that a statue of the Virgin Mary – standing in the shade of a roadside grotto, some twenty feet up a steep, rocky hill – had spontaneously begun to move. As word spread and the media picked up on the story, people flocked to the statue in their thousands. Many came simply out of curiosity; many more to gaze upon it, hold quiet vigil and pray. In the weeks and months after the first sighting, as many as a hundred thousand people made this pilgrimage.

At the same time, there came a spate of reports of more moving statues and other unexplained occurrences from around thirty different Catholic religious sites across the length and breadth of the country.

One of these was in Rathdangan, a tiny village built on a crossroads in the foothills of the Wicklow mountains. The village pub sits on one corner of the crossroads, a small shop and post office on another. A local newspaper article dated 20 September 1985 describes a lonely area that was changed overnight. Between five and six hundred people gathered beside the village hall, where raised on a stone plinth, wearing a painted blue shawl and gazing beatifically down upon the assembled crowd stands the statue of Our Lady of Rathdangan. The journalist, Tony Murphy, reports: 'I heard one young man say to his friends in a West Wicklow accent – "Look, she is moving all the time and her hands are going up and down. She has been doing that all night." His friends didn't seem too convinced.'

Then, as suddenly as it had begun, the whole affair was over. The crowds dwindled, then disappeared. The media lost interest. The Catholic Church remained cautiously neutral and so it was left to psychologists and sociologists to unpick it all, arriving at various competing theories on what has become known in Ireland as 'The Year of the Moving Statues'.

It was the following summer, during a family holiday visiting relatives, that ten-year-old Kate and her two brothers and sister were taken to see the Rathdangan statue by their mother.

Kate was, it's fair to say, painfully unimpressed. 'It was a statue. I didn't care. It was just a dull family trip.'

I meet Kate in a trendy cafe – lots of avocado on the menu – near to her home in Dublin's suburbs. In fact, I arrived before the cafe opened and so waited outside as Kate walked up the pavement towards me, swinging her arms high, punching at the air with each quick stride. She's small, looks much younger than her forty-one years and has an urgent energy about her. When we finally sit down together, she folds her arms tightly. She'll hold herself in this way for much of the time that we speak, and I sometimes have the sense that she is seeking to comfort herself. 'I've never gone back,' she says. 'I've never looked anything up on it or gone back to see it. I've never wanted to.' It's not only apathy that I'm detecting in her voice. There's a resentment, too. She speaks at pace, in an accent that to me sounds strongly Irish but that she describes as 'half and half' from her childhood growing up in London – just one of the things that would contribute to her feeling like an outsider for much of her childhood.

When I was a mental health nurse my relationship with people on the ward, and with their families, was pretty clear-cut: I was part of a team offering treatment – and hopefully kindness, encourage-ment and support. In meeting people to write this book, my role feels less clearly defined. I mention this because as Kate's story becomes difficult for her to tell, and the tears gather in her eyes, I'll feel oddly paralysed. The distress of strangers is complicated, isn't it? We can choose not to see it.

We choose so much of what we see: That statue is moving. That family next door are doing just fine.

The adult world

Kate's mother, Brigid, was born and raised in the Irish town of Blessington, County Wicklow. A beautiful place but with nothing much to do. Her mother's imagination and ambitions stretched beyond her small-town life. She was a hugely energetic, motivated person, and also deeply caring.

So in her early twenties – in the mid-1960s – while still single, she packed her bags and moved to London to train and work as a nurse.

A psychiatric nurse, in fact.

Kate's insights into this period of her mother's life come largely from her discovery of the diaries and journals that Brigid kept during that time. For Kate, reading them conjured up a vibrant young woman with a normal and happy social life, with friends and hobbies and all the concerns of a student nurse. Her mother played tennis, thought about how to wear her hair and how to dress, where to go on weekends and with whom.

The person in these journals felt so removed from the person that Kate knew.

'I'd love to read them,' I say.

'We got rid of everything,' Kate explains. 'I wish we'd kept things like that now.'

It was during her nursing training that Brigid met Kate's father, a fellow psychiatric nurse who had himself immigrated to the UK from the West Indies. They married shortly after qualifying and moved into rented accommodation on a council estate in the London borough of Sutton.

Kate was the second child, arriving two years after her much doted-upon elder brother. 'I don't think my mother liked me very much,' Kate says with a sudden and disarming honesty. 'I think I wasn't what she imagined a daughter would be.' There's a lot to unpack in that – and a lot that Kate doesn't want recorded here. In part, at least, she believes her mother saw her as competition for her father's attention.

This was another side to Brigid's personality. For all her kindness, there were also her occasional and surprising outbursts of jealousy. Kate's earliest childhood memory stretches back to when she was four years of age. Her mother had picked her up from school and Kate was chatting exuberantly about a teacher she liked. She can't now summon the whole memory, but what she can remember – won't ever forget – is the way her mother's shadow fell across her. 'If you like your teacher so much,' she said coldly, 'go live with your teacher.'

When Kate was five years old her sister was born, and three years after that came her younger brother. He was still a toddler in Brigid's arms when, during that family trip to Rathdangan, she insisted that the whole family gather around her for photographs in front of the statue of the Virgin Mary.

It had so far been an unhappy holiday for Brigid. They were in Ireland to visit her sister and nieces, but she was convinced – wrongly, in Kate's opinion – that her sixteen-year-old niece was flirting with her husband. All of that was swept away in the presence of the statue. While her children shuffled around, bored,

Brigid was in awe. She took dozens of photographs that day – used up the entire roll of film.

Kate quietly curses and shakes her head.

'She felt something special there,' she tells me. 'I remember her being excited. And tearful, too. She felt that something was really happening.'

It's easy enough for me to imagine a version of this story in which Kate's father, a qualified psychiatric nurse, was alert to early warning signs and sought appropriate help for his wife. He might have become concerned straight away, when back home in London after the holiday Brigid had the photographs developed and grew obsessed with them.

Only it didn't look like an obsession to begin with. It was just the one photograph of the statue, framed and put up on the wall by the kitchen window.

It was Kate and her siblings who first noticed how much time their mother spent looking at that photograph. She talked about it a lot as she cooked and busied herself in the kitchen. She talked about how the Virgin Mary was looking at her and could really *see* her. The way the light fell across the statue's face; that clearly meant something. And the way that she was smiling.

The more Brigid looked, the more she saw.

'What's for tea, Mum?' Kate was ten years old. Maybe the statue was doing strange stuff. The world is full of magic, right? Even if Kate didn't quite believe it herself.

A few months later and it was no longer just one photograph. There were several copies. Brigid was never without them. She kept one in a book with her at all times. She had more in her bedroom. One of the photographs had some sort of mark on it, from the flash of the camera. Brigid was certain that this light was shining down on her from the statue and that it meant she had been chosen.

She waved the photograph inches from her husband's face. 'Look, you can see,' she shouted. 'You think I'm imagining things? Well, see for yourself. Look at the photographs. There's evidence.'

He must have realised she was unwell. Only he wasn't listening. He was shouting, too. Not about the photographs but about her accusations.

Brigid had grown convinced that he was having an affair – and perhaps he *was* having an affair – but she couldn't possibly know that. So he was calling her paranoid.

Listening to this argument, Kate, who was now eleven and a bright young girl who worked hard at school, realised that she'd never thought of her parents as being two separate people before. Never thought of them as being distinct from each other, with their own separate histories and hopes and expectations. But they were separate people. And they hated each other. Her tears caught her by surprise, as did the startling sound of breaking glass.

In his rage, her father threw a glass mug. Brigid flinched out of the way and it smashed against the wall. Now she was convinced that her husband wanted to kill her.

Over the following days, she hid the kitchen knives. She put most of them in the attic, carried the few she needed for cooking around with her.

At night-times, she crept into the bedroom that Kate shared with her younger sister, locked the door and made up a bed for herself on the floor between them. 'I don't trust him,' she whispered. 'We can't trust your father.'

Mistrust is contagious. The children began to dislike their father, avoid him, fear him. Yet still I imagine a version of this story where he finally sought help. It might be professional pride on my part. Something clearly wasn't right, and if he had only seen it – *and he must have seen it* – he could have done something.

'Either he didn't understand or he didn't want to deal with it,' Kate tells me.

She has no intention of trying to put herself inside his head, describing him only as an 'absence'.

One day, he was simply gone.

Everything that followed would pass unnoticed by the adult world.

Everyone goes somewhere

Drift hypothesis is a term used in social epidemiology. It refers to the downward social movement of people with long-term mental illness and is one way of explaining a noted concentration of mentally unwell people in lower social groups. But it doesn't fully explain this picture. A counter-argument, which we have discussed already, is the social causation thesis. This makes the case that the extra difficulties and stressors endured by people living in financial hardship are likely to have a causal relationship with mental ill health, as well as contributing to poorer overall outcomes.

Either way, there can be no doubt that so-called mental illness tracks poverty and inequality extremely closely.

Brigid opened the front door to the man from Sutton Borough Council. His tone was serious and insistent. 'You've not paid your rent,' he said plainly. 'We're taking this property back. You don't live here any more.'

Kate was standing behind her mother in the doorway. She can still picture this man. His neat, dark beard. His crumpled suit and overcoat.

Brigid tried to protest but the man cut her off. There was to be no room for discussion. 'You're to pack one case of clothes for yourself and one case each for your children. You're leaving today.'

Kate remembers the surge of panic, the confusion. She remembers placing her Sindy doll in a suitcase. They had never been homeless. It didn't occur to her that people could end up without a place to go. She knew that she wasn't allowed her things any more, but she knew they were going somewhere. 'Because everyone goes somewhere,' she tells me.

And they did. To begin with. They were 'temporarily relocated' a few miles away – given a one-bedroom council flat, with no outdoor space, for a family of five. The children were forced to move to new schools in a deprived area. It was a horrible, frightening time. 'Obviously my mother wasn't well,' Kate says quietly. 'But obviously nobody realised she wasn't well. I don't know if that would have made a difference, but nobody realised. And then this thing took over.' They stayed in the one-bedroom flat for an entire year; a year characterised by sibling rows and abusive neighbours and the sickening feeling that at any moment things could get even worse. Then, following a series of administrative errors with Brigid's housing benefits, there was another knock at the door.

This time they were evicted onto the streets.

'There must have been warnings,' Kate acknowledges. She knows that they wouldn't have been made homeless without some sort of official process: letters, phone calls, visits. The problem, she explains, was that her mum could no longer seem to organise herself. She couldn't think ahead, couldn't plan from one day to the next. Life was something that was simply happening to her.

This gradual deterioration in Brigid's organisational skills and volition might be seen in retrospect as the tightening grip of 'schizophrenia'. But her children had no way of knowing this. So let's forget the benefit of hindsight and stay with a thirteen-year-old girl squashed into the back of a taxi, surrounded by plastic carrier bags of hastily packed clothes. Her younger brother is tired and grumpy, and clambering around on her lap. Her sister sits weeping in the middle. Her elder brother presses his jaw against the cold window and stares aggressively into the night. He's angry all the time now. He stopped bothering going to school a long time ago and their mother said nothing about it. When he and Kate fight, which they do often, it's with feet and fists.

Brigid is sitting up front. She's explaining to the taxi driver in a mildly posh and affected voice that it doesn't make any sense because she has enough money, it just came in late, but if he can get them to a hotel for the night, she'll sort out everything in the morning, no doubt.

Except this is the third hotel that will send them away because Brigid doesn't have a credit card to secure the room deposit.

The driver glances into his rearview mirror at Kate and her siblings. He switches off his meter. Kate is grateful to this day. That night he would drive them around South London for hours.

They were finally offered a dormitory room at a YMCA, where they spent the next two weeks. Kate doesn't remember exactly how it came about that her mother then made the decision for them to move to Ireland and be nearer to their relatives, but she remembers travelling on the overnight ferry and arriving in Arklow – a small commuter town on Ireland's east coast, where her mother's remaining family lived. And she remembers arriving at the tiny two-bed terraced house. It was freezing and dark. The plumbing

didn't work. There was a hole in the roof and the ceiling was black
with mould. The carpets were damp, too. Kate placed a bucket
beside her bed. When it rained, the water fell in loud fat drops.

Everyone goes somewhere, and they came here.

The outsiders

*Who's the family arriving from London with no dad? You know their
mother has been seen walking about there in town talking and
laughing away to herself. And she was telling all them in the post
office that she's Mary's chosen one, can you believe it? And you know
where they're all living, do you? All five of them! Can you believe it?
Where do they sleep, poor things? Oh, but you can't get involved, can
you? Sure, it's their own business. Don't they look odd though, too?
They do though, I'm just saying is all. Is that from the father, do you
suppose?*

Arklow was a town where everyone knew everyone. At their new
school Kate and her sister were immediately branded outsiders.
They were labelled the Addams Family. She believes they stood out,
in part, because they looked different to most people in that community. Remembering this today, she self-consciously touches her
hair and face. 'We were just really small and pathetic-looking,' she
says. 'We were just young-looking and small-looking and odd-
looking. And all probably a bit antisocial-looking.'

On three separate occasions kids from the neighbourhood
smashed the front windows of their house with stones.

Finding it impossible to integrate, Kate and her siblings hid
away behind their locked front door, and watched as their mother
continued to sink deeper into a world of her own imagining.

Within weeks of arriving in Arklow, Brigid had fallen out with
her extended family by accusing them of plotting and scheming

against her. These were the uncles, aunties and cousins that might otherwise have been on hand to offer support. Now they turned their backs, perhaps too embarrassed or ashamed to acknowledge the circumstances that this mother and her children found themselves in. Or else, Kate suggests, they simply had too many of their own problems to contend with.

Brigid started drawing maps. She owned an old atlas and each day would sit with it open in front of her for hours at a time, drawing on the pages, making hundreds of cryptic notes. She was hearing voices constantly. And constantly she responded to them, whispering beneath her breath.

'Who are you talking to, Mum?'

'None of your business! None of your business. Leave me to my work.'

And it was work. Important work.

With her atlas, and in communication with her voices, Brigid was fixing war zones. She was preventing global conflicts from breaking out. She frequently commented on newspaper stories. 'That's my work. Oh, you see, my work is happening. It's happening!'

It can be too easy – perhaps even tempting – to separate what we might perceive as a person's psychosis from any meaningful motivation on their part. To see madness simply as madness, rather than risk it becoming tangled up in the complicated business of our humanity. Except this was the same woman who could never walk past a homeless person without offering help. It was the same woman who used to take care of stray animals – leaving out food for a fox and its cubs, and even once bringing home an injured pigeon so that it wouldn't starve. And now she was working tirelessly to make the world a better place for all of us. This was her vocation. It was why she got out of bed in the mornings. At times, Kate recalls, she looked frightened and distressed by what she was hearing but she could also be happy, excited, filled with a sense of purpose. Her motivation, if not its execution, was indisputably noble.

On the flip side, her obsession with the vital work she needed to do was drawing her further away from the immediate needs of her four children. In Kate's words: 'We were living in conditions of great hardship. She found comfort and reassurance in her visions and voices.'

For a long time, Brigid's strange behaviours were – to her children, at least – a small, secondary frustration next to the bigger backdrop of poverty. They were desperately poor and, like many people who are barely surviving in the benefits system, they were also trapped in cycles of spending that only made them poorer. Brigid would use the electricity money for food, then get behind on electricity payments. She sold her wedding ring. She sold whatever she could. She was stuck buying overpriced, poor-quality food from the local corner shop because they offered her a tab. Frequently, the family were without heating and electricity. At least once their water supply was cut off.

Here's the thing: it only takes a couple of paragraphs to describe the day-after-day of such a life. But to live the day-after-day is a whole other story. Such poverty, Kate impresses upon me – in bursts of rapid speech that leave no room for interruption – such poverty has a dull and aching monotony: every Tuesday is like every Friday; every June like every September. Life is thinking and worrying about food and how long it will last, and thinking about the bills and when they are due, and worrying about whether or not the rent has been paid. It is television and arguments and restless sleep, or lying awake, worrying. And that was as much as it could be. There was nothing else. There was no variety, no change, no family events, no holidays. Birthdays came and birthdays went. They were miserable, they were depressing, they were hard.

At the end of each school year, Brigid would sell her children's textbooks, then struggle to find the money to buy them again. Kate frequently took time off school rather than get into trouble for not having the right books or other classroom equipment, which they could never afford. More troublingly, her youngest brother started school two years late because Brigid kept him at home, unable to organise his education. He only started after the authorities threatened to prosecute, and it occurs to me that they might instead have offered to help.

'People leave you to yourselves,' Kate says. 'They assume that if you have problems someone else is dealing with those problems. It's the same if you see someone talking to themselves in the street. You assume they're okay. Yes, they're odd. You mightn't want to be their friend or get to know them or chat about the weather. You might avoid standing next to them. But you're not going to think: "That person's talking to themselves, that's a problem, let's do something about it." And if that was your attitude to everyone, that would be awful as well.'

'Would it?' I ask.

She shakes her head. 'I don't know. I don't know. Some people are actually in treatment, or their families are trying their best, but the symptoms are still there. Probably family are the only people who really know.'

Fifteen-year-old Kate pushed aside her homework and took a new sheet of paper.

Dear Dad

But now what?

What if she put on paper the things that were happening: how she would stir in her sleep and wake to see her mother across the darkened room, staring at the walls, whispering incessantly at the plug sockets. And how during the days Brigid drifted from room to room like a ghost, unreachable in her own inward-gazing world. How she verbally lashed out at her children, throwing hurtful accusations at them – declaring that Kate was a prostitute who sold herself to her teachers.

If Kate wrote about how she could no longer remember the last time her mum had simply hugged her or said 'I love you'; if she wrote to her dad that they had no money, that they desperately needed money; could he please send them money? If she wrote it all down in a letter, then what? She had no idea where to send it. And even if she could find an address for him, what if he chose to throw the letter in the bin, abandon them again? Wouldn't that be worse?

No, she wouldn't write to her father. What about speaking to a teacher at school? Might they be able to do something? They had to know something wasn't right. But then what if they sent someone round? Someone from social services who would look at them and sneer and judge. Someone who would step off the road and through the front door and immediately be in this room. This dingy and bleak little room. Kate and her sister doing their homework at the table; her elder brother sitting in front of the blaring TV; her mother talking to herself on the stairs.

And what if they took her mother away? What if they locked her up somewhere? What if they separated Kate and her siblings and they all ended up in care? What about her little brother? Wouldn't that be worse?

No, she wouldn't ask for help. This was their secret. They would bring themselves up, drag themselves up if necessary. Day after day, month after month, year after year. And every night, every single night without fail, Kate raced through the rosary and asked God to make it stop. 'Please let this stop. I will do anything. Just let her wake up normal. Just make her be normal. Make this stop.'

An awful thing to do to a human being

Against the odds, Kate excelled at school and was shepherded into higher education – which at the time was free – by teachers who recognised her potential, even if they failed to see her needs.

She was easily the strongest student in her year group. In fact, for all the enormous trials they faced at home, in the classroom all four siblings shone. Her elder brother would take longer to find his path, though. Kate describes him as the most intelligent of the bunch, but he was also the most exposed to and affected by their life behind closed doors. And so he stayed at home, slumped in front of the TV, as Kate took daily commutes to Trinity College Dublin, where she studied medicine. He turned up the volume to drown out their mother's shouting.

Brigid left the house once a week to collect benefits from the post office before locking herself away again. 'She was in her room all the time,' Kate tells me. 'There was a period where she just locked the door and stayed in there, shouting. It wasn't even whispering any more. She was shouting. She had no life now.'

Kate was a good way into her studies when, flipping through a psychopharmacology textbook in the university library, she chanced upon a chapter on schizophrenia – something she had always presumed to mean 'split personality'.

Her pulse quickened. She recognised her mum on every page.

I imagine Kate rushing home to tell everyone. I imagine their questions, a door opening, the shaft of light, a sense of possibility.

It didn't work out that way.

'Very good, Kate. It has a name. That doesn't change anything.' Her brother was still watching TV.

After so many years he refused to believe anything could ever change. In truth, Kate didn't believe it could either. They had lived with this since childhood. It had been the last ten years of their lives. The youngest knew nothing else. It was normality.

And there was another complication. Somewhere amid the confused feelings that now swarmed around their household was guilt. If this thing had a name, if other other people had it too, if there were treatments – why had they done nothing sooner?

'You were children,' I suggest.

'We were still like children,' Kate insists. 'Even when we were twenty, twenty-one, twenty-two, we were still like children. I went to college like I went to school. I didn't have other exposures. I grew up in this bubble. I didn't even know other people. College and home was the same as school and home. We just weren't mature.'

I begin to say that this makes sense to me. How could it be any other way? Frankly it's impressive, more than impressive, extraordinary that—

I hit upon something impenetrable.

We're not really in conversation at the moment. We're in the same place, sitting across a table from each other. I'm making my notes and ostensibly Kate is speaking with me, but at the same time it's as though I'm not here. When I do speak, I come up against what I suspect to be the same psychological shutters that she pulled down to keep the world at bay for so many years. She's started so she'll finish, but I'm not coming in, and I'm certainly not allowed to say anything to make her feel better. That wasn't the deal.

Kate first went to the GP on her own. There was no possible way to convince her mum to go. Brigid hadn't been to the doctor for many years. Her paranoia meant she refused to let anyone examine her. She wouldn't even go to the optician, despite suffering from increasingly poor eyesight. She wasn't about to let some stranger shine a light into her eyes. God only knows what that might do.

In fact, this represented one of Kate's main worries. Her mum was getting older and though she didn't smoke or drink alcohol, she certainly wasn't living the healthiest of lifestyles, cooped up in a damp and mouldy bedroom, doing no exercise, eating the plainest of foods. If she were to get physically unwell – blood pressure, cholesterol, whatever – nobody would know.

Kate wasn't here to talk about that, though. She was here to tell the GP about her mother's behaviours. She told as much as she felt able to in order to convince the doctor that her mum needed help – though this doctor added the caveat that when a person has been chronically unwell for so long, often treatment doesn't make an awful lot of difference. Then there were technicalities to deal with. She had to sign paperwork to say that her mother wasn't capable of making her own decisions, and that it was in her best interests to be admitted to hospital for treatment. Because Kate wasn't the eldest, it needed to be countersigned by another relative. She needed the support of her siblings. Her elder brother was extremely resistant. He didn't agree that their mother needed to be treated. He figured Kate was interfering. The arguments stretched long into the nights.

'It's not nice,' Kate says, turning away from me. 'It's not a nice thing to do. You are taking the right away from someone to make their own medical decisions. It's an awful thing to do to someone. It's a huge thing to do to a human being. Especially when this has been going on for so long and you haven't done anything about it. It's an awful thing to do to someone. It's really an awful thing to do. It's a terrible thing to take away somebody's rights from them.'

The greatest fear was that they might be putting their mother into a hospital that she would never come out of. It was the most difficult decision of their lives. But they made it.

All four of the siblings went to the GP and signed the paperwork.

If they loved you

Brigid was collapsed in an armchair, hardly able to open her eyes. She hadn't put her top set of dentures in. Her mouth was dry and sticking together as she attempted to speak. 'Oh, the doctors have given me something, Kate,' she managed. 'I shouldn't be here. This is a terrible mistake. I want to go home.'

People used to joke about Newcastle psychiatric hospital in County Wicklow. *If you're not careful you'll end up in Newcastle*, they would say. It's one of those places. People assumed nobody really went there. Only the crazy people. An *other people, not us* kind of place. That was Kate's impression, anyway.

Walking through the grounds wasn't so bad. All the greenery and trees. Once inside, though, Kate felt scared for herself, and scared for her mum.

She went to take hold of her mum's hand, but hesitated. She felt so guilty, so remorseful, so sorry for what she had done.

Things improved, and surprisingly quickly. In part, Kate puts this down to it simply being a new environment, with greater stimulation and more clearly defined boundaries. In recent years, as she and her siblings were getting busier with their own lives, and crucially as even the youngest was able to take care of himself, there had been little left to tether Brigid to reality. She was getting forgotten and in her isolation had free rein to venture ever deeper into her delusions.

We're all a bit madder when we're on our own, aren't we?

Kate used the time when her mum was in hospital to do something she knows they should have done years earlier. She reported their landlord to the Department of Health.

In the ten years they'd lived in that house he'd refused to fix anything, denied anything was wrong with the property, boasted sardonically that it was in fine condition, that they didn't build them like this any more. The Department of Health inspectors disagreed. He was forced to make substantial improvements throughout.

Meanwhile, Kate and her siblings searched for somewhere new for them all to live. Somewhere that would accept social welfare payments.

'Vulnerable people like we were are always sympathised with in the abstract – but not when they become real.' This is how Kate explains it to me. 'Many nice, caring, normal people were involved in evicting my family, making us feel like outcasts, stepping away from us, ignoring us. We were let down by social services, school teachers, doctors, councils, landlords, family and mental health services. Not because of individuals – these were all nice people, many with families – but by the systems that surround them.'

They did find somewhere new to live. It wasn't easy but they found somewhere. A warm, clean, spacious bungalow that, when she was released from hospital, Brigid could call home.

If you didn't know the circumstances, weren't privy to the history, you might overhear it and think nothing of it. To Kate, though, it was huge. She was heading out to university and her mum was in the living room, watching a daytime TV show about makeovers. That in itself was unusual. The TV was always on but Brigid never sat down to watch it. For her, it was something to keep her children subdued, to stop them from fighting.

Or else it was another means for her to telepathically communicate with a world that nobody else could see.

Her admission to hospital had only lasted for a couple of weeks – long enough to establish her on antipsychotic medication and refer her to a community team. She was still drowsy. Still sleeping a lot of the time. She looked up from the TV and spontaneously addressed her daughter. 'So I learnt today that if you're putting on lip gloss and you want to look elegant you should just put it on your bottom lip. It's less tarty than if you put it on both lips.'

That was it. She turned back to the programme.

It was a snippet of normality. That's what Kate calls it. To take a little bit of information from the world and retell it to someone – no, not just to anyone, to her, to Kate.

And Kate realised that after so many years she had never expected to hear her mum saying something so small and wonderfully ordinary again. There were other snippets, too. The time Brigid asked for a Joni Mitchell CD, and then for a book she'd heard about. Specific things that revealed interests returning to her life. Kate is cautious not to overstate the significance of this. Brigid remained largely withdrawn. She tired easily and became bored by things quickly. Medication, Kate discovered, was no magic cure. 'It just softens the edges of the paranoia – but leaves a drooling, sleepy, lonely person behind.' She believes her mother was still talking to the walls, still hearing voices, but that this was more contained, no longer the whole of her.

Then came the evening that they went into Dublin together to watch the Vienna Boys' Choir. By this time Kate was working as a junior doctor and had enough money to take her mum on trips and weekend breaks. Kate remembers this particular trip because upon entering the National Concert Hall she felt embarrassed by what she'd chosen to wear. All around them were women in high heels and glamorous dresses and Kate felt childish in her flat shoes with flowers on them, her embroidered brown skirt that suddenly seemed impossibly nerdy.

'God, Mum,' she whispered. 'I dress like a child.'

Brigid smiled, kindly. 'You can dress any way you want. As long as you're happy with it,' she said.

And telling me this today, Kate's eyes are awash with tears and she is beaming. Because that's something a mother might say to a daughter, isn't it? It's something someone would say if they loved you.

It was a few days after Christmas that Brigid called an ambulance for herself because she was struggling to breathe. She was taken into hospital. Her whole body was aching. She was tired, jaundiced, had a cough she couldn't shake. She was sixty-two years old.

They began running tests but this was still the holidays. There were fewer senior staff on duty; everything was taking longer than it ought to. Brigid needed a catheter and Kate remembers how much this distressed her. She was convinced she was going to die.

'Look after your brothers when I go,' she told Kate on New Year's Eve.

'You are so dramatic!' Kate laughed. 'You're not going to die.' But she could see how frightened her mum was and so she hugged her. And kissed her. It was a strange moment for both of them. 'Because we never hugged,' Kate tells me. She's hugging herself. Her voice cracks a little as she speaks. 'We didn't touch. As far as I can remember I never hugged or kissed her. Probably when I was really young. But we weren't affectionate.'

Brigid rolled her eyes, hugged her daughter back. And Kate knew she was happy. She knew she was happy that someone had given her a hug.

The scans revealed that the tumours were everywhere: her lungs, ovaries, liver, everywhere. She was going into total organ failure. Brigid was sick for one week. Then, with all of her children at her bedside, she passed away.

After living through such a huge challenge for more than half her life, such a death felt dismissive to Kate. To merely die of something so common and almost routine as cancer seemed unnatural. Kate believes her mother deserved a greater death.

'It's still ridiculous to me,' she says. 'It's still absolutely ridiculous that she could get cancer after that bizarre, horrible, shitty life. That you have three years of almost scratching something back to normal. And then you die of cancer. It's ridiculous. I still feel—' She stops, shrugs, can't find the words.

In the decade that has passed since Brigid's death, Kate's feelings towards her have moved from the anger, fear, frustration and confusion of her childhood towards an admiration. In the most cruel of circumstances, she did what she could. A single mother, penniless, persecuted, surrounded by visions and voices that nobody else could see or hear – and living in communities that refused to see or hear her – she kept four children together, kept a roof over their heads, put food on the table.

'No matter what else she was like,' Kate concludes, 'this was my mother.'

Delusions

'WHEN ONE PERSON SUFFERS FROM A DELUSION, it is called insanity. When many people suffer from a delusion it is called a religion.' So wrote Robert M. Pirsig in *Zen and the Art of Motorcycle Maintenance*. It's a quote that came to mind as I thought about all of those people in Ireland, flocking to the statues of the Virgin Mary, believing them to have spontaneously sprung to life. As far as I'm aware, those people weren't collectively deemed to be mentally unwell.

I'm not about to argue that there was no difference between them and Brigid. I believe that there was. I believe there are substantive differences between whatever fleeting thoughts those thousands of people may have entertained, which had been normalised – indeed, encouraged – by their communities, and the more intensely held beliefs of Brigid; beliefs that she couldn't shake even as her community isolated and ostracised her. Those two mindsets aren't the same. They do, however, have important things in common. And I would argue that the Year of the Moving Statues is an illustration, as if it were needed, that all people, including ostensibly 'sane people', have a staggering capacity to believe in nonsense.

We humans are not, on the whole, especially rational creatures. Our minds are filled with prejudices, superstitions, misremembered details, lies we've told ourselves and opinions-held-as-fact. And once we do believe something we tend to hold on to it tightly, regardless of its veracity. As the historian James Harvey Robinson observed: 'Most of our so-called reasoning consists in finding arguments for going on believing as we already do.' In fact, a study conducted at Ohio State University showed that people spend 36 per cent more time reading an essay if it aligns with opinions they already hold.[1] If that statistic rings true, you should give the rest of this chapter your full attention. If it doesn't, maybe skim-read it.

As we have come to expect, deciding when a person's unusual beliefs constitute a 'mental illness' is far from an exact science. Psychiatry's definition of delusions changes with each update of the DSM, and in a surprising twist DSM-5 did away with the need for a belief to be false in order to be considered delusional.

That may sound counter-intuitive but I'm inclined to agree that it was a sensible move. Imagine that you're convinced your partner is cheating on you. There's no evidence for this, and what you perceive to be evidence seems very strange to other people. The way that clouds move across the sky indicates that the affair is occurring, and your partner's secret lover is sending you taunting messages through TV programmes. You are certain of all this despite your partner's desperate efforts to demonstrate their fidelity. In fact, the more they try to convince you that they are not being unfaithful, the more certain of it you are. When they agree to stay at home with you rather than go out with friends, it's just another way that they're toying with you. Each time you leave the room, or even turn away, your partner and their lover are in secret communication.

Now suppose that it turns out your partner actually is having an affair. Would the reality of that mean that you're not delusional? Have you been cured?

I suspect not.

In DSM-5, delusions need only be 'fixed beliefs that are not amenable to change in light of conflicting evidence'.[2] That's a broad definition, and one that may describe more of our beliefs than we'd care to admit.

At the same time, some beliefs are so bizarre in their content that they do stand out from the crowd as being especially broken. I am thinking again about the journalist, Molly, and her belief that she had committed a number of serious and highly improbable crimes, that newspaper headlines were referring to these and that MI5 were tracking her through a camera placed in her womb. And the soldier, James, who became convinced that the army had selected him for a secret mission, and later that he was a messianic figure. Similarly, Brigid believed that she had been chosen by the Virgin Mary to carry out important and supernatural work in the world. Again, the proof of this work could be seen in the newspapers.

Those beliefs are obviously not commonplace. Though if I'm being perfectly honest, I wasn't shocked by them either. Anybody who has worked at the sharp end of mental health services will be familiar with such narratives. Psychiatric nurses in the US mightn't come across too many patients who believe that MI5 (or, I suppose, more 'likely' MI6) is tracking them through secret listening devices, but we know they work with a great many people who are convinced that the CIA or FBI are doing so. Depending on where we are in the world, the Virgin Mary may be replaced by the Prophet Muhammad or some other religious or important cultural figure, but save for the name and a few other changes, unerringly similar pictures emerge across all cultures. Indeed, given the unfathomable myriad of beliefs that human beings are able to concoct, one of the most surprising features of delusions (at least, the delusions that bring people to the attention of psychiatric services) is how few themes there seem to be.[3] We'll return to this in a moment. First, let's consider what is by far and away the most common theme: persecution.

'Two distressing beliefs are at the heart of persecutory delusions: harm is to occur to me and other people intend it.' This is the observation of Daniel Freeman, a Professor of Clinical Psychology at the University of Oxford, who specialises in the study and treatment of persecutory delusions. 'Paranoid thoughts like these are extremely prevalent,' he tells me. 'And that's because we're always making decisions about whether to trust people or not. So it's not surprising that often we get it wrong.'[4] His research suggests that between 10 and 15 per cent of people, and maybe as many as a third, regularly experience paranoid thoughts. We are, Freeman believes, only now really beginning to acknowledge and talk about this. He also suspects – though the data isn't there to test – that we may be becoming more mistrustful as a society, and that related to this we are feeling increasingly unnerved, anxious and frightened.

As an unnerved, anxious and frightened man who devotes too much of my time to worrying about what other people might think of me – and frequently assuming the worst – I'm sympathetic to that view. Though again, I come back to my point that believing people are talking unkindly about us is qualitiatively different to believing that people have placed a microchip in our brain in order to control our thoughts.

If nothing else, the first scenario is at least possible.

'Having an erroneous mistrustful thought is, of course, not the same as having a persecutory delusion,' Daniel Freeman agrees. 'But it is not unrelated. It might be analogous to feeling mildly down in mood compared to a depressed episode. Yes, they're different but it's not completely unrelated processing that's going on. What you are looking at with paranoia is probably a greater presence of the different causal factors. Greater sleep disturbance, greater levels of worry, lower self-esteem, greater trauma history, greater reasoning biases, all further along the spectrum.'

Some of Daniel Freeman's most revealing work has focused on the relationship between persecutory delusions and the *neurosis* of excessive worrying. (Neurosis, in this context, refers to mental distress characterised by anxiety, depression or other feelings of unhappiness that do *not* involve the radical loss of contact with reality that defines psychosis.)

Worry, Freeman suggests, brings implausible ideas to the mind, keeps them there and increases the distress that they cause. And it turns out that levels of worry in people with severe paranoia are similar to those levels seen in people diagnosed with 'generalised anxiety disorder' – the archetypal disorder of worrying about stuff.

Now, I suspect that most readers won't be too surprised by that revelation. It stands to reason that people who suffer from terrifying beliefs are also going to worry about them. Yet this simple observation has been somewhat neglected by the mental health research community, at least in part because of a tradition of conceptually separating 'neurosis' and 'psychosis'. So if a bizarre psychotic delusion is present, the focus of psychiatric study – and by extension, psychiatric treatment – tends to be on that, while overlooking any associated 'neurotic distress'. The problem with this, according to Daniel Freeman, is that neurotic thoughts such as extreme worry are not only *present* alongside delusions but may also *contribute to* and *sustain* delusions. 'Certainly, excess worrying plays into paranoia,' he tells me. 'It means that we give a lot more headspace to the paranoid thoughts. It also makes us elaborate the content, so ever more unlikely things are thought about. And, crucially, it inflates our estimate of how probable it is that our fears are going to actually happen.'

That final point needs a bit of unpacking. How does simply thinking more about something increase our belief that it will occur?

Well again, we human beings are far from rational creatures and a cognitive bias that affects all of us – whether we're experiencing psychosis or not – is an unconscious tendency to overestimate the likelihood of something happening if it comes more readily to mind. This can be influenced by how recently a memory, opinion or worry was formed, as well as how unusual or emotionally charged it is. It's why nobody wants to go swimming in the sea after they've just watched *Jaws* (and presumably why nobody wants to watch a movie ever again after they've just watched *Jaws: The Revenge*).[5]

'More than anything else, what I see in people with severe paranoia is that they've withdrawn from life because of their fears,' Freeman explains. 'They don't want to encounter other people so they spend more time alone, and then worry takes over their lives completely. We sometimes believe that we can solve a problem by worrying about it. But it's an inefficient and unhelpful strategy because it skews our judgement.'

I suspect there's a lesson in there for most of us.

In 2015, Freeman and his colleagues conducted a study in which people experiencing persecutory delusions were offered a psychological therapy that focused purely on techniques to identify and reduce 'worry thinking styles' rather than challenging delusional content. 'It's a nice way in,' he says, 'because people can recognise that worrying makes things worse without having to get into a dispute about how true or not their worries are.'

The results of this trial were encouraging. It was shown that people's levels of distress came down, and so too did their levels of belief in their delusional thoughts.[6] That's not to say that such an approach will be right for everyone, or indeed that it would help with the many other distressing experiences we've come to associate with so-called schizophrenia. But for some people who are consumed by false beliefs of persecution, this might represent a useful chink in their delusion's armour.

Modern psychiatry's interest in delusions tends to be focused on their presence or absence rather than their content.

This is especially so in the US, and is a criticism levied against his own profession by Joel Gold, Clinical Associate Professor of Psychiatry at New York University School of Medicine. 'Delusions, like all thoughts produced by the mind, have meaning,' he writes.

> Yet psychiatry today is not inclined to this view, has no interest in why different brains choose different delusions, and is simply interested in eradicating the psychotic symptom. This is curious. Our patients take great interest in the content of their delusions – is there any reason to think they shouldn't? Most of us take our own thoughts seriously and a basic premise of psychiatry is to think about thoughts. When we listen closely to what our patients are saying, paying attention to psychotic and non-psychotic thought with equal consideration, we foster the therapeutic alliance, and stronger alliances yield better therapeutic outcomes. The fact that delusions mean something to our patients is reason enough for them to mean something to us.[7]

Amen to that.

It's also true, as I mentioned earlier, that when we scratch beneath the surface of delusions common themes invariably emerge.

It's because of this that delusions are sub-categorised. We've discussed the most common category, persecutory delusions, as experienced by over 70 per cent of people suffering a first episode of psychosis. The next most commonly seen are *grandiose delusions*, where a person comes to believe that they have extraordinary powers, wealth, influence or fame. Other types of delusions include: *delusions of reference*, which is the belief that events in the environment – such as people's gestures or TV programmes – are directed at the delusional person or have a special significance to them; *erotomanic delusions*, when an individual believes – falsely and unshakably – that another person is in love with him or her; *nihilistic delusions*, which involve the conviction that a major catastrophe will occur; and *somatic delusions*, involving a preoccupation with health, bodily function or organ failure.

I find it surprising that the two most common themes – persecution and grandiosity – are so different from each other. Hiding away from the world because it's out to get you seems the polar opposite of believing you have special powers and are untouchable.

Speaking to me from his psychotherapy practice in Lower Manhattan, Joel Gold suggests otherwise. 'They're intimately connected,' he argues. 'If one feels persecuted, there's an inherent grandiosity to that. If the CIA believes that I'm carrying around some secret which puts me at great risk – that's grandiose.' It chimes with what we learnt from Molly, doesn't it? When she was at her most poorly she didn't believe herself to be some unremarkable crook; she was Britain's Most Wanted. We can also look at this the other way around, starting with grandiosity. 'Let's be concrete,' Joel suggests. 'If you think you're Christ then crucifixion is not very far around the corner. You have that inherent sense of risk. People will want to bring you down, call you a false prophet.'

It's an intriguing observation, though for Joel Gold the more compelling similarity – and one that may connect all of the delusions that I've mentioned – is the unique way in which they concern themselves with our social world and with the threats that we face within it. Gold's theory, as developed with his brother Ian Gold, an Associate Professor of Philosophy and Psychiatry at McGill University in Canada, is that delusions stem from a breakdown in a mental capacity that helps us to navigate the dangers of social living. He calls this the 'suspicion system'.

'That we need to negotiate and survive the social world is just a fact,' Joel Gold argues. 'And it's none too easy, right? It's quite a challenge. It pays to be vigilant to potential threats.'

The key word here is *potential*. There's no point being vigilant to a threat that's already materialised and done its damage. No, we need to anticipate danger in order to avoid it. This requires us to be sensitive to any number of environmental and social warning signs, some of which will be highly ambiguous and speak only to our gut instinct. Consider the scenario that Joel and Ian Gold offer in their book *Suspicious Minds*, in which they ask us to imagine that we are walking through a dark forest or a bad neighbourhood late at night:

A slight rustle behind you is most likely dry leaves pushed around by the wind – but could also be the careful steps of someone preparing to spring at you. A successful cognition system for threat detection must be able to draw your attention automatically, motivate you to start thinking hard (if unconsciously) about what the sound might mean, and move you to act if action seems warranted. In addition, the motivation that is produced by a threat system like this should suppress competing impulses temporarily, until the threat has passed. Responding to a sound that might signify danger requires full attention even if it turns out to be a false alarm. Being vigilant in this way means that you will have to act on the basis of uncertain information; but when it comes to wolves in forests or assailants in alleys, it's better to err on the side of caution. What we call 'fear' is one such cognitive system: an automatic, unpleasant, highly effective mechanism that commandeers our full attention for the purpose of self-preservation.

The 'suspicion system' doesn't only concern itself with the kind of threats that might endanger our lives. According to the Golds' theory, it's looking out for us at all times, in our every social inter-action. Triggered by a gesture, a facial expression or the subtlest change in a person's behaviour, it's the hunch we have that a friend is lying, that our partner is going to be unfaithful or that our boss intends to offer the promotion to someone else.

Such things matter at a deep, evolutionary level. What we're talking about is nothing less than our ability to produce and pro-vide for offspring and to maintain our safety and status in the tribe. It's imperative that our brain be on the lookout for any risks to these things in order that we can take preventative action – and far better to suffer the stomach lurches of a few false positives than to turn down the sensitivity of this radar and suffer the far worse consequences of a significant threat going undetected.

We don't, for the most part, go through life like startled rabbits. After the initial jolt of fear in the dark alley we're not *forced* by our brain to run away. In this respect, the 'suspicion system' can be seen to fit into a well-established model of cognition known as 'dual process reasoning'.[8] What I've so far described is System 1 thinking, which is rapid, intuitive and unconscious. It's an alarm bell sounding in an ancient part of our brain. Then System 2 kicks in. This is our controlled, thoughtful, conscious reasoning. It's slower to get started because it requires a lot more effort, but once up and running it's able to carefully appraise the threats detected by our flighty System 1, and examine them for veracity.

'Nah, it's all right,' says System 2. 'That's not a terrifying spider. It's just the harmless top of a tomato.'

(Or for the lycopersicoaphobics among us: 'That's not a terrifying tomato. It's just the harmless top of a spider.')

I've simplified this for brevity, but central to Joel and Ian Gold's theory is that delusions flourish when this extremely useful – indeed, necessary – system of threat perception breaks down. Our unconscious suspicions grow overly sensitive, finding threat where there is none, while our reflective reasoning fails to properly hold this in check. If we subscribe to their theory then it makes perfect sense that ideas of persecution are the most prevalent in delusions because they are closest to the normal function of suspicion. Paranoia is nothing more than suspicions that cannot shut themselves down, a broken form of threat detection; whereas grandiosity, according to this theory, is a broken form of threat response.

Remember, the whole purpose of our 'suspicion system' is to alert us to potential danger so that we can take action to avoid it. As we heard from Daniel Freeman, the most common way people do this is to shut themselves away from the world. When this isn't possible, however, different survival strategies may be necessary – and if we can't make ourselves small to hide from a perceived threat, well, we might just need to make ourselves look big in order to send that threat packing. It's a strategy seen ubiquitously across the natural world. In the uniquely complicated societies of human beings, though, flexing our muscles and puffing out our chest isn't always going to cut it. So we do something else. As Joel and Ian Gold observe, when under pressure, we often subtly exaggerate our importance in order to gain the upper hand. It's true, isn't it? We talk ourselves up, make certain our virtues are on display. Occasionally we lie about how we really think and feel in order to protect our social status. And with a bit of effort, we can even convince ourselves that those lies are true. But enough about every Facebook post ever written.

Grandiosity, it seems, may be nothing more than an unregulated version of a normal social coping strategy.

From this perspective, we can begin to frame each of the commonly seen delusions as either a breakdown in the system designed to detect social threats or a maladaptation in the way we respond to these perceived threats. Even something as strange as *delusions of reference* begins to make more sense when we consider that a healthy 'suspicion system' needs to be alert to the subtlest of cues in our environment – a glance, a gesture, an overheard conversation – which may be referring to us with malicious intent. Misfiring or unmediated suspicion is inevitably going to find such references in ever more unlikely places.

It's a speculative theory and there are many, many others out there. I've focused on it because of how it helps to make sense of some of the environmental causes of psychosis and so-called mental illness that we discussed earlier in this book. You'll recall that being a victim of child abuse or being separated from a parent in childhood or moving schools several times during adolescence or being an immigrant or being bullied or living in more densely populated areas each increases the risk of a person becoming psychotic. What do such experiences have in common?

Certainly, each brings with it levels of stress. But so do many other life events which do not increase a risk of psychosis. No, what they each share is that they evoke fear. And according to Joel and Ian Gold, it's a particular kind of fear, demanding heightened and protracted vigilance.

The victim of abuse or bullying will be anticipating and trying to avoid future assaults. In the case of a parent leaving, we've lost an important figure of protection and must be more watchful for ourselves, while perhaps unconsciously (or consciously) striving to avoid further abandonment. Each time we move school everyone is a stranger, and so we must learn quickly who is safe and who is not. Same if we're an immigrant. And the more densely populated our environment, the more strangers we have to fear and be suspicious of. Delusions may be the cost of maintaining highly stressful levels vigilance, in order to stay safe.

Now, dear reader, if you'll indulge me, here's a quote from my own novel, *The Shock of the Fall*:

> I have an illness, a disease with the shape and sound of a snake. Whenever I learn something new, it learns it too. If you have HIV or Cancer, or Athlete's Foot – you can't teach them anything. When Ashley Stone was dying of Meningitis, he might have known that he was dying, but his Meningitis didn't know. Meningitis doesn't know anything. But my illness knows everything that I know. This was a difficult thing to get my head around, but the moment I understood it, my illness understood it too.

My protagonist is getting to grips with the curious relationship between his psychosis and his knowledge of the world, with each influencing the other. He's talking from a personal perspective but if we examine trends over time we can also see that delusions are shaped by the very same forces that determine the worldview of the period.

This was demonstrated nicely in Slovenia, where the medical records of psychiatric patients who had been admitted to hospital between 1881 and 2000 were reviewed. It was found that religious delusions, which were prevalent at the start of the twentieth century, took a steep decline between 1941 and 1980, during which time Slovenia was part of the communist dictatorship of Yugoslavia. The government suppressed religion and the less people engaged with it, the less frequently it featured in delusions. From 1981 to 2000 – after communism crumbled and Slovenians were once again able to worship – religious-themed delusions re-emerged.[9]

Joel Gold isn't surprised. 'For a symptom characterised as a break from reality, psychosis keeps remarkably up to date with the outside world,' he remarks. 'Whatever culture one is steeped in will show up. For much of history, religion was the central organising theme of people's lives. Since the mid-nineteenth century, as religious commitment has become more optional for many, we've seen a corresponding decrease in delusions with religious content.'

What he has seen a marked increase in, however, is what he calls 'the *Truman Show* delusion', in which the delusional person believes that they're being constantly watched via hidden technology for the entertainment of others, as was the case for the protagonist played by Jim Carrey in the 1998 film.

In his clinical practice, Joel Gold began to see increasing numbers of people with this delusion from the early 2000s. 'I'm not suggesting that the *Truman Show* delusion comes entirely from the movie or the technology therein,' he says. 'But it would be, I think, very unlikely for such great social shifts – tectonic shifts in technology, in social media, in the surveillance state – for these changes not to have a major effect.' Most disturbingly, he believes, the radical change to our social lives that technology has brought about over the past twenty years is not only shaping the content of delusions but is likely a causal factor in itself. In much the same way that urban environment increases risk of psychosis, so too might the fact that we're all jammed together online.

'People spend more time on Twitter, Instagram and Facebook and are less happy,' Joel Gold explains. 'I think it's bad for people's mental health, full stop. So if you have someone who's predisposed to psychotic illness and they become familiar with social media – they mightn't even be on it, but simply be aware of its existence – it plays right into longstanding persecutory ideas of "people are watching me". Well, people *are* watching us. If you're on that spectrum, maybe with a hyper-sensitive suspicion system, that's going to have a real impact.'

I'm fairly sure it's illegal to write an essay on the subject of delusions without quoting the psychiatrist and philosopher Karl Jaspers (1883–1969). 'Since time immemorial,' he wrote, 'delusion has been taken as the basic characteristic of madness. To be mad was to be deluded.'

It's a quote that pops up everywhere. Yet it seems to me that the longer we spend sitting with these strange thoughts, the less mad they appear and the more clarity they offer. None of us is immune either. Our many biases and fears ensure we're all at least a bit deluded. Since time immemorial, delusions have been a basic characteristic of people.

But what about other unusual experiences? Delusions needn't visit in isolation. Another long-established theory is that these strange narratives are nothing more than an attempt on the part of the believer to make sense of other anomalous experiences.[10] 'She was hearing voices constantly,' Kate told me about her mother.

'And constantly she responded to them, whispering beneath her breath.'

Brigid's experience didn't stop with the things that she believed. She could also hear something.

We should think about the voices in our heads. First, though, it's time to address something that may unite more people with a diagnosis of serious mental illness than anything else.

Chemical Treatment

YOU MAY REMEMBER AMIT. I talked about him at the beginning of this book. He was the first of many people that I have forcibly medicated against their will.

It seems a bit strange to write that sentence now. My days of working in acute nursing are a long way behind me and I find it hard to see myself as part of a Control and Restraint team, injecting chemicals into people who desperately didn't want those chemicals injected into them. Of course, I did so legally, and in what I believed were the best interests of our patients. I was working alongside some of the kindest and most caring people I have ever known and we were motivated by trying to help, not harm. At the same time, I can't help but feel a bit conflicted about it all.

Amit isn't a white person. So having crossed paths with psychiatry in the UK, his odds of being in this situation were considerably higher than that of the white patients on the ward. In fact, a recent independent review – ordered by the government – revealed that black and minority ethnic psychiatric patients are four times more likely than white patients to be sectioned in hospital under the Mental Health Act. They are also ten times more likely to be placed on treatment orders upon their discharge from hospital. These community orders require patients to remain on strict medication regimes, attend assessments and agree to other living arrangements or risk being returned to the ward.[1] This significant imbalance in how these powers are used contributes to what is often referred to as 'the over-representation of black and minority ethnic people in mental health services'.

A better name for it is institutional racism.

One of the chairs of the review, Steve Gilbert, has spoken about his own experiences as a black man navigating the psychiatric system. 'Most of the disparity in decision making isn't conscious,' he explained.

I've not come across staff that are racist, but I have come across staff who were ignorant about the issues that affect people from black African Caribbean communities. When we think about the decisions that are made, more often than not you're perceived as presenting a risk if you're a young black African or Caribbean male – as opposed to someone who is white [. . .] I've got a really loud voice, but that can be misinterpreted as me being aggressive. But it gets a bit loud when I'm scared or anxious.[2]

Psychiatry's problematic relationship with black people stretches back at least as far as the days of slavery in America, when a slave might be diagnosed with 'drapetomania' – the name given for the so-called mental illness of trying to flee from captivity.[*]

In his book *The Protest Psychosis*, Dr Jonathan Metzl charts the unsettling and cynical connection between black civil unrest in the United States in the late 1960s and early '70s and rates of schizophrenia diagnosis. He argues that it was from this time that black men began to be disproportionately categorised as schizophrenic, with the idea developing among some in the psychiatric community that the beliefs and feelings inspired in African Americans by the 'Black Power' movement were themselves symptomatic of psychotic disorder. In other words, a legitimate struggle of an

---

[*] Yes, you read that right.

oppressed people was conflated with a psychiatric illness. The drug companies saw a marketing opportunity in this and, as Metzl reveals, prominently depicted images of 'aggressive-looking black men' in their advertising materials for antipsychotic medications.

That level of extreme institutional racism isn't apparent in today's mental health system either in the US or in the UK. Yet there's still clearly work to be done. One problem area in the UK relates to staffing. In the aforementioned recent mental health review it was acknowledged that clinical psychologists are dispro-portionately white and female, and do not necessarily have train-ing in 'transcultural therapy' or a deep understanding of specific issues relating to racism and discrimination. The result is that peo-ple from black and minority ethnic communities are less likely to engage in – or to be offered – the therapies that may reduce a need for hospitalisation.

So there are a multiplicity of complex reasons why people such as Amit are more likely to find themselves detained and medicated than white people who are experiencing the exact same kind of psychotic symptoms.

Now let's turn our attention to why we medicate anybody (irre-spective of their race or cultural background) and consider what exactly it is that antipsychotic medications do.

First, it will be useful to know a little of the history. It turns out that 1952 was a fairly monumental year for psychiatry. Not only – as we learnt earlier – was it the year that the American Psychiatric Association published its first edition of the DSM, but it was also in the spring of this year, at Sainte-Anne Hospital in Paris, that the prominent French psychiatrist Jean Delay, together with his assis-tant, Pierre Deniker, began injecting their most disturbed psy-chotic patients with a newly synthesised chemical compound called chlorpromazine. This was the single biggest moment in the history of modern psychiatry and its repercussions continue to influence the lives of almost everyone diagnosed with schizophrenia today – and, for that matter, people diagnosed with a whole host of other mental health-related problems, such as major depression and anxiety.

Chlorpromazine, the world's first so-called antipsychotic medication, has an interesting family tree. As part of the phenothiazine family of chemicals, we can trace its lineage back to 1876 when a German chemist, Heinrich Caro, synthesised a phenothiazine derivative for use as a cost-efficient dye in textile production. He called this dye methylene blue.* In the decades that followed, phenothiazine and its derivatives would serve a number of surprisingly varied functions ranging from insecticides to medications for the treatment of parasitic worms, and, in 1949, an antihistamine that was first administered clinically by an innovative surgeon in the French navy, Henri Laborit.

Laborit – who in a wonderfully French way was also a philosopher and man of literature – had theorised that the newly discovered antihistaminic properties of the phenothiazine derivative, promethazine, could be used on his surgical patients to treat post-operative shock: a horribly distressing and sometimes deadly condition characterised by rapid heart rate, cold sweats and a precipitous drop in blood pressure that is itself caused by the body's excessive release of histamine, which can occur in response to major wounds. Upon successfully using promethazine in his surgery, Laborit observed that in addition to its usefulness as an antihistamine it also calmed his patients down, appeared to have

---

* It was yellow.†

† JOKE. It was blue.

painkilling properties and resulted in them experiencing what he poetically described as a 'euphoric quietude'.[3] Researchers at Rhône-Poulenc, the French pharmaceutical company that had synthesised promethazine, responded by creating an even more potent compound, which is how we arrive at chlorpromazine.

Again, it was surgical patients who got the first taste of this new drug. French surgeons reported enthusiastically on its powerful anaesthetic qualities and how it induced a 'twilight state' in patients.[4] Henri Laborit then mooted the idea that chlorpromazine might also be useful in psychiatry and when Jean Delay and Pierre Deniker put this theory to the test the results were astonishing. Patients who had been gripped by severe agitation and fear appeared suddenly calm, subdued and untroubled. The use of chlorpromazine spread rapidly though the asylums of Europe in the 1950s, with the same effects reported everywhere. A British psychiatrist, Dr Anton-Stephens, described the drug's main effects as 'somnolence' and 'psychic indifference', which were useful in 'quieting disturbed behaviour'.[5]

Of course, none of this should be confused with these patients being somehow brought back to their 'normal selves'. Far from it. Here's how Delay and Deniker described their newly medicated patients at the time:

Seated or lying down, the patient is motionless on his bed, often pale and with lowered eyelids. He remains silent most of the time. If questioned, he responds after a delay, slowly, in an indifferent monotone, expressing himself with few words and quickly becoming mute. Without exception, the response is generally valid and pertinent, showing that the subject is capable of attention and of reflection. But he rarely takes the initiative of asking a question; he does not express his

preoccupations, desires, or preference. He is usually conscious
of the amelioration brought on by the treatment, but he does
not express euphoria. The apparent indifference or the delay of
the response to external stimuli, the emotional and affective
neutrality, the decrease in both initiative and preoccupation
without alteration in conscious awareness or in intellectual
faculties constitute the psychic syndrome due to the
treatment.[6]

The term 'psychic syndrome' is, I think, extremely pertinent
here. It was evidently the impression of Delay and Deniker that
whatever syndromes their patients presented with prior to being
given chlorpromazine were, in effect, replaced by another powerful syndrome of the drug's own making.

That's not to say that patients would never have chosen this new
syndrome in preference to the terrors they endured beforehand. In
many cases, I don't doubt that they would have done (though it's
difficult to find first-person accounts from this time). I'm simply
highlighting the fact that the choice wasn't between 'psychosis'
and 'wellness'; it was between 'psychosis' and a 'twilight state'.

It's also important to note that nobody described chlorpromazine as an antipsychotic – or talked about it having antipsychotic
qualities – during this initial period of its use. Delay and Deniker
called it a 'neuroleptic' (the suffix from the Greek *lepsis*, 'sei-
zure'). This caught on in much of Europe. In the United States,
the more blunt description of 'major tranquilliser' was preferred.
The prevailing view, as captured by the American psychiatrists
Joel and Charmian Elkes, was that psychotic symptoms persisted
but that 'patients became quieter, less tense, and less disturbed
by their hallucinations and delusions'.[7]

It wasn't until 1961 that chlorpromazine (by this time marketed in

Europe under the trade name Largactil and in the US as Thorazine) was first described as an 'antipsychotic medication': a term coined by the Canadian psychiatric researcher Heinz E. Lehmann, considered by many to be the father of modern psychopharmacology.[8] The term gained traction and is now ubiquitously used to describe chlorpromazine and the generations of similar drugs that have followed it. Among critics of psychopharmacology, this is deemed to be a profoundly misleading description, as indeed is the term 'antidepressant'. We'll come back to the reasons why in a bit.

It was also Heinz E. Lehmann who came up with the term 'extrapyramidal' to describe what are some of chlorpromazine's most common and most debilitating side effects. These include acute dyskinesias and dystonic reactions, tardive dyskinesia, akathisia and akinesia.

Those will be unfamiliar words to many readers. Luckily you're in the presence of a qualified nurse, so allow me to shed some light.

Dyskinesia is involuntary rhythmic contraction of large muscle groups. *Tardive dyskinesia* involves this happening to the tongue, lips and face, resulting in clenching of the jaw and uncontrollable chewing, lip-smacking motions. *Dystonia*, in contrast, is a prolonged contraction of muscles causing extreme stiffness, abnormal posture and difficulty moving properly. *Akathisia* is also a disorder of movement but describes a horrible feeling of inner restlessness. People experiencing this find it hard to sit still and often fidget constantly, pace, and rock back and forth. *Akinesia* is pretty much the opposite, as characterised by a partial or complete inability to move. Collectively, these symptoms are called Parkinsonism as they are essentially the same symptoms that we see in Parkinson's disease.

On psychiatric wards, where gallows humour is culturally embedded, these symptoms came to be known as the Largactil Shuffle (or Thorazine Shuffle in the US). There's a cruel irony to the fact that many of the symptoms stereotypically associated with madness – shuffling, rocking, pacing and so on – are actually caused by psychiatric medication.

I also think there's a cruel irony to the term 'side effects'. To my mind, it would be fairer and more honest if we talked instead about a drug's *desired* and *undesired* effects. The reason why is captured by something James (the soldier) told me. You may recall that chlorpromazine was the drug that he was given when he first went to hospital. He'd suffered horrendous experiences caused by this treatment and told me that, on balance, he believed that the side effects far outweighed the usefulness.

I'd argue that any effects which *far outweigh* the others aren't *side effects*: they're the *main effects*. And let's not forget that some of the so-called side effects of chlorpromazine – such as intense drowsiness and the twilight state – were clearly its intended functions when it was being developed for use in surgery. It feels a little bit like cheating to try to have it both ways.

For better or worse, chlorpromazine completely altered the landscape of mental healthcare across the globe.

By 1964, around 50 million people had taken it.[9] It was the standard treatment for so-called schizophrenia for decades. In the UK, it played a significant role in allowing for the closure of the large, long-stay asylums, paving the way in the 1960s and '70s for government policies of deinstitutionalisation and a move towards the smaller hospitals and community-based mental health services that we have today.

By the time that I first walked into one of these community-based wards in the late 1990s, the use of chlorpromazine and other so-called 'first-generation' antipsychotics (such as haloperidol, which we predominantly used for the 'rapid tranquillisation' of distressed and aggressive people) was on the decline, replaced by what are called the 'second generation' of antipsychotics.

There was a lot of optimism (or at least a lot of optimistic marketing material) when these newer drugs were developed, not because they were deemed to be more effective as treatments but because they seemed to cause fewer extrapyramidal effects. However, in time it became clear that they did still cause some of these effects – such as tardive dyskinesia – as well as a whole raft of their own unpleasant and dangerous symptoms, including, most commonly: anxiety, increased saliva production, drowsiness, indigestion, restlessness, constipation, light-headedness, nausea, stomach pain, stomach upset, dizziness, dry mouth, fatigue, headache, trouble sleeping, vomiting and weight gain, leading to related complications such as diabetes and heart disease.

We've come across several of these second-generation drugs in this book already. They include all of the drugs that Clare's son, Joe, was tried on – and that she ultimately holds responsible for much of his physical and mental decline prior to his death.

So this is where things get complicated, because if we take another story, such as that of the journalist, Molly, then we get a far more positive interpretation of these medicines.

People with first-hand experience of taking psychiatric drugs differ profoundly in their views about them. Such was the reflection of Jim Read, who, after twenty years of involvement in psychiatric service user and survivor movements, concluded: 'For every person who says their life has been ruined by psychiatric drugs, there is someone who believes they have been saved by them, and many more who just don't know, who have been taking them for years and wonder if their lives would have been better or worse if they had been free of them.'[10]

A part of me is tempted to leave this discussion at that. Because if you or people you care about are taking psychiatric drugs and finding them helpful, then they're helpful. That's great! I have no interest in changing your mind.

Likewise, if you've taken these drugs and believe that they've harmed you then that's because they've harmed you. I've seen those lists of 'side effects' in action. I'm not going to pretend that isn't harm.

There will never be a consensus of experience. And yet what does seem to unite the overwhelming majority of people who use psychiatric services is that they are *offered* these drugs. 'Psychiatric drug prescriptions are still the prevailing answer to the multitude of problems that cause people to seek or receive professional help,' writes Jasna Russo, a mental health researcher who has personal experience of being treated in the psychiatric system. 'When in contact with mental health services in the Western world, hardly anyone can get around being offered, prescribed or forced to take psychiatric medication.'[11]

That's certainly been the case for the people I've encountered in writing this book. And it's for this reason that I wish to reflect a little more on what we currently understand about these chemicals: how they help us, how they harm us, and how they shape so much of our current thinking about mental health and illness.

This discussion comes with the caveat that even the basics are confusing. Psychopharmacological research is a dark art. In 90 per cent of trials comparing different second-generation antipsychotics, it was found that the results favoured the sponsoring company's product. This leads us to some bafflingly paradoxical outcomes: *olanzapine beats risperidone, risperidone beats quetiapine, and quetiapine beats olanzapine.*[12] Reading this stuff can feel like falling into an Escher painting.

Also, more than sixty years on from the discovery of chlor-promazine we still cannot say with certainty how antipsychotic drugs actually work.* We need to start somewhere, though, so let's start with the grandaddy of all psychiatric theories: the dopamine hypothesis.

Antipsychotics were in use for more than a decade before it became clear that they blocked dopamine signals in the brain. It was precisely their success (or at least, perceived success) in treating so-called schizophrenia that resulted in some suggesting that schizophrenia was caused by excess dopamine signalling in the first place.[13]

Few now think it's as simple as that, and early iterations of this dopamine hypothesis have been largely abandoned. But it's a theory that frequently gets reinvented, and most of the researchers and academics that I've interviewed believe that dopamine plays a crucial role in the experience and pharmaceutical treatment of psychosis. This raises a number of questions. How exactly would high levels of dopamine manifest as a psychotic experience? Also—

'Shhh. Listen. Can you hear that noise?'

I'm once again interviewing the schizophrenia researcher Professor Robin Murray at the Institute of Psychiatry in London. He's interrupted my questions about dopamine because he's suddenly become aware of a strange noise in his office.

I can hear it, too.

'That hissing noise?' I ask.

'Yes.' He looks perturbed. 'What do you think that is?'

For the briefest second, I wonder if we should be worried. Then

---

* Here, I use the term 'work' to mean how they exert their desired effect of reducing distress by reducing the intensity of psychotic experience.

I settle on it being the air conditioning system.

'Dopamine is a neurotransmitter that does several things,' Professor Murray explains. 'Most simplistically it can be seen to relate to pleasure. That's the reason why people take drugs like amphetamines, which increase dopamine. But dopamine also plays a role in cognition. The higher your dopamine levels, the more salience things around you will seem to have. If you have too much dopamine in your brain and you hear that same noise, the air conditioning or whatever, it will stand out, feel important and significant to you.'

Human beings aren't terrific at paying attention to more than one thing at a time (actually, no animals are) and the theory goes that dopamine plays a central role in directing our attention to the more personally relevant things in the world around us, allowing us to filter out the constant deluge of irrelevant things. Dysregulation in our dopamine system may therefore result in all manner of commonplace events – the sound of the air conditioning, or a stranger crossing the road in front of us, or a song being played on the radio, or the argument that our neighbours are having, or a newspaper headline, or the movement of the clouds across the sky and the feeling of the breeze on our face – arriving in our consciousness with the same feeling of them being worth paying attention to that we experience when our phone buzzes in our pocket or a fire alarm goes off. And it stands to reason that if all these stimuli shared that same quality of salience to us, we would begin to infer they must all be somehow *about* us, leading to either mania (*I must be very important*) or paranoia (*the world is out to get me*).

What does all this have to do with antipsychotic medication?

Well, as I said a moment ago, we know that one of the main effects of these chemicals is that they block certain dopamine receptors in the brain. They may therefore diminish this 'aberrant salience' and so negate any related psychotic thoughts.[14]

That's an intuitively neat theory but there are holes in it. I've already alluded to a major one. Recreational drugs such as ecstasy, amphetamines and cocaine cause veritable fireworks displays of dopamine in the brain, but they don't (on the whole) make us question our sanity. They make us feel marvellous.

Now, becoming addicted to stimulants can – over time – lead to a paranoid psychosis. However, this presents a paradox because by the time things descend to that stage, stimulant drugs tend to cause a relatively meagre dopamine release compared to those initial exhilarating blasts. 'For the dopamine hypothesis,' write Robin Murray and his colleague Paul Morrison, 'this dissociation between the acute versus the chronic pharmacology of stimulants is problematic.'[15]

It's perhaps also worth stressing here that dopamine theories of so-called schizophrenia do not exist in isolation from the psychological and social causes I've discussed previously in this book. We know, for instance, that stressful life events such as child abuse and migration result in increased dopamine synthesis. Furthermore, the stress and anxieties that so often accompany psychotic beliefs are likely to result in a further release of dopamine, as are any frightening consequences of psychosis such as compulsory hospitalisation.[16] This observation points to another problem with the dopamine hypothesis. What little hard evidence there is for raised dopamine activity in people with acute psychosis comes from small studies comparing their brain activity with groups of 'healthy controls'. But there are likely to be many more differences between these two groups of people than just the presence or absence of psychotic thinking – not least that the participants with psychosis are more likely to be agitated, stressed and anxious. It's conceivable that this, and other factors not specifically linked to psychosis, may explain away any differences in dopamine levels.[17]

At best, current theories seeking to directly link so-called schizophrenia and dopamine are overly simplistic.

However, we do know that the blockade of dopamine – as caused by antipsychotic drugs – is certainly linked to the extrapyramidal effects which I described earlier. This has led some academics to arrive at the rather more grim interpretation that antipsychotics seem to work precisely *because* they cause Parkinsonism – not just the physical symptoms as seen in the worst of the so-called side effects, but also the psychological symptoms of Parkinson's disease such as emotional blunting, diminished interest and apathy.[18]

'It's important to understand', explains Dr Joanna Moncrieff, 'that the drugs we prescribe for mental health conditions are mind-altering substances. They change people's behaviour and thinking by inducing states of intoxication rather than reversing an underlying medical disease.'

You will remember that we met Joanna Moncrieff earlier when talking about the many possible causes of so-called mental illness. She's an expert on psychiatric drugs and is concerned that there are a lot of misconceptions about them – certainly among the public, but also among many of the professionals who prescribe and administer them.

When discussing antidepressants and antipsychotics, she draws a parallel with alcohol. 'We have the expression in English of drowning your sorrows,' she says. 'So we recognise that if you take a drug like alcohol it will change your emotional state. We don't think that alcohol is acting on the biochemical basis of depression when we say that, though. We just recognise that the characteristic effects of alcohol will inevitably change whatever it is that you're currently feeling.'

It's for this reason that Dr Moncrieff (and many others) don't much like the terms 'antidepressant' and 'antipsychotic'. They argue that the names give the misleading impression that these chemicals somehow specifically target depression or psychosis in the brain, in the same way that antibiotics target the micro-organisms responsible for bacterial infection. If that was your impression, then you have been misled.

Antipsychotics, Moncrieff suggests, are better conceptualised as a 'blunt instrument'. They suppress a whole range of mental activity, which just so happens to include things like delusional thoughts.

'It's a really difficult situation for patients,' she acknowledges. 'A really, really difficult situation because that suppression of symptoms can be so helpful. But the price people pay is often just terrible. They're horrible drugs. And it's even sadder in a way when people get used to them, so they've forgotten that they're horrible. And you think: *my goodness, you don't remember what it was like to have strong emotions and to feel things, do you?* Because often that's what people say that they hate when they first start taking them. The emotional numbness. But then they get so emotionally flattened that they stop caring about being emotionally flattened.'

One of the most shocking fears about antipsychotic drugs is also one of the most difficult to investigate. This is a bit technical but it's also important, and isn't a part of the mainstream conversation about antipsychotic medication – even though virtually every expert I have spoken with has acknowledged it as a legitimate concern.

It relates to something called 'dopamine supersensitivity'. To make sense of this, it's vital to understand that antipsychotic drugs don't actually reduce synthesis of dopamine in the brain. Rather they block a type of dopamine *receptor* in the brain – called a D2 receptor – which means that the dopamine can't exert its influence. But we now know that when people take these drugs over a long period of time, the brain responds by growing more of these receptors at the sites where they've been blocked.

The first problem then occurs when people do decide to stop their medication, because not only are the dopamine receptors no longer being blocked but there is a proliferation of them for the dopamine to get to work on (hence 'supersensitivity').

For this reason, we might conclude that once started on these drugs people would be less vulnerable to relapse if they stayed on them, and that may well be true, but the story gets more complicated. As the D2 receptors proliferate, antipsychotics naturally become less effective at blocking them. We know that many people who faithfully take their drugs as prescribed – including taking ever higher doses to compensate for dopamine supersensitivity – still suffer from relapses. The crucial question this raises is: Does taking antipsychotics over long periods eventually render a person *more* prone to relapse than if they'd *never* been prescribed the drugs in the first place?

'The problem is that we can't test for this,' explains Professor Robin Murray. 'It would require a study where one group of people with psychosis is randomised to *not receive* medication. No ethics committee would allow it. First presentation psychosis. You couldn't not give them antipsychotics.'

The decision to medicate people at the first sign of psychosis is partly the result of a cultural shift over the past couple of decades.

Reflecting back to when I first started nursing, there's no doubt that we handed out a lot of medication, but if someone was on their first admission to hospital it was common practice to wait a couple of weeks before giving antipsychotic drugs. The idea was to see whether, in a safe environment, things settled down of their own accord.

That doesn't happen any more. Successive government cuts to mental health services mean that today people need to be considerably more disturbed before being offered a bed, and at the other end of the process are discharged much sooner – often before meaningful recovery.[19] The pressure for turnaround is such that there simply isn't the time or money available to wait and see. 'If you need to get people out quickly, what can you do?' asks Dr Joanna Moncrieff. 'You have to drug people up to the eyeballs. That's the only option you've got. And that happens.'

Such practical constraints are compounded by a theoretical notion that the longer a person's psychosis is left untreated before they commence medication, the poorer their long-term outcomes will be. Part of the thinking behind this claim is a throwback to the discredited view of schizophrenia as a deteriorating brain disease – a theory sustained by evidence from MRI scans showing that people who have lived with a diagnosis of schizophrenia for many years suffer from a reduction in cortical volume (literally a shrinking of the grey matter). The conclusion reached was that over time schizophrenia caused progressive brain atrophy.

But of course, the people who had their brains scanned not only had a diagnosis of schizophrenia, they'd also been taking antipsychotics for many years.

In what is perhaps the most chilling of the many contradictions and bitter ironies we've so far encountered, we now know – in part due to primate studies, in which macaque monkeys were given prolonged courses of both first- and second-generation antipsychotics

– that this reduction in brain tissue is the result not of schizophrenia but of the medications used to treat it.[20]

Notwithstanding these developments, concern about prognosis being worse the longer psychosis goes untreated was a major force behind the establishment of 'Early Intervention in Psychosis' services across the United States, Canada, Australia and much of Europe since the turn of the millennium.[21] In the UK, this also shapes clinical practice policies (known as the NICE guidelines, from the National Institute for Health and Care Excellence), which press for adults with a first episode of psychosis to start treatment in early intervention services within two weeks of referral.[22]

To be clear, I'm not about to criticise that guideline. If someone I loved was losing touch with reality then I'd want them to be seen by a specialist immediately, because I don't doubt that I'd be scared shitless.

From my professional contact with early intervention teams, I also know that they don't reach straight for the medicine cabinet in every situation and that the treatments they offer include a growing range of talking therapies. That being said, these services are also operating under significant pressures. They're obliged to get people started on treatments rapidly and the quickest and easiest form of treatment will always be the prescription pad.

'Then there's the misplaced consensus that people must keep taking medication to prevent relapse,' continues Moncrieff, 'though if you look at the antipsychotic trials, there's actually no consistent definition of what "relapse" even means. A lot of the time they're looking at relatively trivial increases in symptoms, which might be better termed as a slight symptom fluctuation. It's really, really important that we work out whether or not we're making people more relapse-prone by giving them long-term medication. And I do think it's possible we could be making some people who would just have a few psychotic episodes through their lives actually worse overall.'

————

For all that I have said about the potential dangers and limitations of the so-called antipsychotic medications, my personal view remains that they absolutely do help many people.

When working as a mental health nurse, I witnessed a small minority of people whose lives were positively transformed by them. Sometimes, over a course of days, I would watch someone return from whatever dark and distant place they had been lost. See their relief as the world reformed and took shape before their eyes. See them saved.

That's not romanticising.

I've witnessed this.

It wasn't what I witnessed with Amit, though.

'Do I have to beg you?' he'd asked, when we entered his room.

Even if he had begged, it wouldn't have made a difference. The decision was already made. My hands trembled as I injected him, and continued to shake as I took the used needle and syringe back to the clinic, safely disposed of them, signed his medication chart.

I was the nurse-in-charge of that shift and decided to place Amit on 'close observations' – meaning that every fifteen minutes a nurse would go and check on him to make sure he was safe. I walked down the corridor to his room many times myself, lifting the observation slat on his door, looking inside.

He spent the day lying on his bed, his face pressed into the mattress, weeping.

It feels clear to me that doctors and other mental health professionals need to be much, much more cautious about getting people started on these drugs in the first place. It's also clear to me that, in the words of one academic I interviewed, there's a 'gaping chasm in the evidence for when to stop prescribing'.

That makes sense. The largest antipsychotic studies are often sponsored by drug manufacturers. It should not be surprising that the emphasis has been on when people should start taking these drugs, rather than when they should stop. It may be that mental health professionals need to help people to safely come off antipsychotics much sooner than current habits of practice dictate.

Naturally, there will be some people who will benefit from longer periods on medication, where it is suppressing what would otherwise be a continuous distressing experience for them (and that's without opening the whole other can of worms relating to people who are choosing to repress what would otherwise be a continuous distressing experience for their loved ones). Even in these cases, though, we must be much clearer about what these drugs are – intoxicating substances – as well as their limitations and the potential risks associated with their long-term use.

Among the biggest mistakes health professionals can make is to assume shared priorities. For some people the considerable costs of experiencing psychosis will be preferable to the costs of its chemical treatment.

Now let's consider a phenomenon that all of us experience to lesser or greater degrees: hallucinations.

And let's meet a mental health nurse who hears voices.

THE KEYHOLDER, THE NON-KEYHOLDERS AND THE VOICES

Age 6 I remember my dad, huge and omnipresent in his combats ordering me my first issue of *The Amazing Spiderman*, the simple buzz each week of hearing the letter flap slam shut and the drop on the mat, knowing the next instalment was here. Connection. Protection. Dad gave me his helicopter headset once whilst he was away. I broke it pretending to be him, playing. He looked disappointed but not angry. That sense of disappointment I took and filled the vacuum of his absence with, it threads and binds my memories, it squashes, pinches, flattens me, even now.

> *This quote and those that follow are taken from the interviewee's own reflective writing.*

I'M NOT REMOTELY SURPRISED when Jasper describes his GP from twenty years ago as being 'absolutely lovely'. Throughout my time with Jasper, it's noticeable how he finds the best in everyone. If that's an effort for him, it doesn't show. People are fundamentally decent in Jasper's worldview, and it occurs to me that this must be a useful disposition to have in his line of work. Jasper is a senior nurse with a specialist service, where he works with troubled men whose psychotic experiences have either made them an extreme risk to themselves or else driven them to seriously harm or kill other people.

'He was absolutely lovely,' Jasper tells me, in a hushed, almost reverent tone. 'He was a bit of a hippy. He wore these Hawaiian shirts. He never once talked to me about diagnosis. I never had a diagnosis put on me, ever. And I've never taken meds. I'm not saying they wouldn't have been helpful. But my story is one of recovery without them.'

Another doctor, another day, it's easy to see a different narrative unfolding. It's easy to imagine Jasper receiving a diagnosis of schizophrenia.

He was with his GP to discuss the recommendations made following a psychiatric assessment. It's a fuzzy period in his memory and understandably so. He'd grown extremely paranoid in his late teens and early twenties. His parents were living overseas and he was alone, struggling to pay the bills and keep things together in their family home in the UK.

His father worked for the armed forces and a transitory upbringing on various military bases meant Jasper had no real friends or support in this part of the country. To pay the bills, he was putting in shifts at a meat-packing factory and a local dockyard. Then he'd return to this house. 'It was a huge house,' he recalls, 'a massive old Victorian thing. About a third of an acre of gardens.' He shakes his head, guessing correctly at what I'm thinking. 'It probably sounds very posh. It had a swimming pool at the back, too. But that was completely disused and knackered. It was all falling apart. I slept in my parents' old bedroom, with my single bed pushed right up in the corner. The rest of the room was totally empty and it was just me sitting in the corner of that huge, cold room. And I had these terrible, splitting headaches.'

He avoided looking out of the window because he could hear people in the neighbouring buildings talking about him, spreading rumours. He would catch the edges of their conversations, filling in the gaps with his worst fears. *The Whisperers*, he calls them now – a way of helping to make sense of them, in part for himself, in part for other people. At the time, they had no such name and he'd no reason to think that they weren't entirely real.

Perhaps *think* isn't quite the right word. He had no reason to *feel* they weren't entirely real.

'I'm quite a rational person,' Jasper says, 'and I've often wondered why I didn't employ that same logic when thinking about my voices. Why I didn't reason with myself that there was no possible way I could be hearing people talking in distant buildings. The loose conclusion I've reached is that it's because those experiences were much more emotionally held, as opposed to logically held. The drivers underneath them are far more emotional.'

Jasper's emotional and (at the time) unquestioning relationship with his voices makes a lot of sense to me when considered in the context of when he first started hearing them.

He was six years old.

'A misconception of many people who work in mental health is that a first voice must be this big, pivotal event – and it's not always,' he says. 'For some people it can be. For me it wasn't. I just didn't think anything of it. Children are so accepting of things, aren't they? I had no assumption that this was different, that it was abnormal.'

The voice was Spider-Man. Or, more accurately, it was Peter Parker. Talking about this with me today, Jasper falters and looks away. He's in his late forties, has a wife and three children and a meaningful career. We're speaking at his home, which he and his wife have lovingly renovated themselves. Put another way: he's a grown-up. He's embarrassed to be talking to another grown-up about the depth of his connection with a comic-book character.

'I did have other friends,' he assures me, 'but we moved home a lot. Friendships on military bases always feel so transitional. You form them quickly and they end quickly. Whereas Peter

Parker was consistent. He was older than me and I sort of looked up to him. And I really hooked into the idea of spidey sense. I can't pinpoint exactly when it happened but if there's one stand-out occasion it was at my birthday party. I was either turning six or seven and there was this girl who I quite liked and I'd asked my mum to invite her along. I remember sitting on the stairs, waiting for her. Then spidey sense kicked in: *She's not coming, she's not coming*. And as it happened, she didn't. That's the most concrete memory I have. It was a long time ago.'

Though Jasper refers to this first experience as a voice, I suggest to him that his description of it sounds closer to a feeling or an instinct. A sudden or unbidden thought, perhaps? An intuition? Is that fair?

'It was the sense of knowing something was there but it wasn't as tangible as other things,' Jasper tells me. 'At first it was the sense of a friend. Something or someone who was able to offer a kind of consistency and companionship. It would be wrong to describe it as a thought process, I think, but it was the least distinct of my experiences.'

There was nothing indistinct about the voice that arrived a few years later, when Jasper was nine.

His dad had a posting abroad. His mum was going, too. It was decided that Jasper would remain in the UK and attend a boarding school. He remembers the family discussions about this and also his strong desire to make it okay for his mum and dad. 'I knew that my parents needed me to say that I was happy with the decision, that I wanted to go to that school,' he explains. 'So that's what I told them.'

On the day he was dropped off, Jasper had to be physically held back by a member of staff. His mum was in floods of tears, too. That night, Jasper slept in a dorm with other boarders. He describes a pair of pyjamas made for him by his grandmother, a talented seamstress, whom he adored more than anyone in the world. She had lost the tips of her fingers in an industrial accident. 'She could thread a needle one-handed,' Jasper recalls. 'She was absolutely amazing.' We've digressed for a reason.

It was early morning during that first week. Jasper was awake, lying in bed, still feeling somewhat shellshocked in this unfamiliar new world.

'Time to get up,' she said.

He knew that it wasn't his grandmother, but at the same time it somehow was. And when she spoke – this familiar, caring, compassionate voice – she awoke the same feelings that his grandmother always evoked in him: a certainty that he was loved, that someone was watching over him, that he wasn't alone.

Over the coming years, she continued to speak to him. Always gently, always with kindness.

Did he tell anybody about her?

'No. I never did. To be honest, I never thought to. For me it didn't feel unusual or different. I felt no reason to tell anyone.'

I suggest that he might have if he had thought other people could hear her as well.

We're both mental health nurses, so he knows exactly what I'm getting at. He knows when he's unwittingly found himself subject to an ad-hoc mental state examination.

'If you pinned me down on it, I knew she was internal,' he says. 'One hundred per cent. I knew that she was inside my head and that nobody else could hear her. But when the external ones came, the Whisperers, I didn't tell anybody about those either. Because by then I was completely invested in the experience.'

So something changed for Jasper somewhere. His voices went from being a source of comfort, companions residing within him, guiding him, caring for him, to something profoundly distressing; voices that drifted through open windows, through cracks in the walls, and who hated him.

That change, I discover, came after an event in Jasper's adolescent life. He was in sixth form. Jasper tells me something that he doesn't want recorded here. His reason is out of respect and courtesy for other people. That's fair enough. What's important, I think, are the feelings he was left with. Feelings of shame and regret. Feelings of a lost future that he can never put right or atone for. I tell him it wasn't his fault. Because it wasn't. No blame need be apportioned. These things happen.

'Putting it into that intellectual context doesn't make it right, doesn't make it any better,' he says.

As it happens, I don't agree with him. I think context is everything. But there we have it. Like so many of the good people in this world, Jasper reserves his harshest criticisms for himself.

At first they were the voices of people I knew, heard just out of earshot, down a corridor, outside a door, in a kitchen in a house I was walking by. And then came the voices of people I didn't know, in an office I could see into the window of, of people on trains behind me or at the end of the carriage, of people in the street, all picking at my paranoia, playing on my self-doubt, crushing what esteem I had left.

For the next five years, during which time Jasper completed a degree in history and civil rights movements, these Whisperers were never far away. But neither were they constant.

Jasper talks about a set of scales or a balance: on one side are stabilising factors, on the other are destabilising factors. Though university wasn't exactly a walk in the park, he did find himself in a strong and nurturing friendship group. So life was stable and the voices grew less intrusive and less distressing.

It was in the years after university, when he was living alone in his parents' crumbling house, that the scales tipped too far the other way.

I've already said that Jasper didn't have friends in that part of the country, but he did have somebody. His grandmother. The real one. She lived a few roads away. Jasper wanted to be near her. It was hard, though, because by this time she was suffering from Alzheimer's. They'd play cards together. 'She used to be such a card sharp,' he tells me. 'At Christmas she'd have everybody's money! But now she was forgetting how to play, or it would take her three or four games to remember. My parents were overseas. I'd lost my friendship groups from school and university – and now I was kind of losing my grandmother at the same time. It just all smashed together. And I really, really began to unravel.'

At its worst the Whisperers were constant and unyielding, 24/7. I remember in my early 20's stumbling around a housing estate hearing the Whisperers from every kitchen, every living room, destroying me.

Jasper started getting migraines. He locked himself away, stopped taking care of himself. 'I couldn't even walk down the street to the shops,' he tells me. 'I dreaded going outside.'

Then one morning, he was still in bed, afraid to get up, and exactly as had happened all those years before, his grandmother's voice spoke to him. 'It wasn't the same as before,' he explains. 'It was much, much louder. Like somebody had turned the volume right up on the radio. I don't know whether she needed to talk louder to be heard.'

Though the volume was cranked up, it was still the same caring voice. Somebody was watching over him. Once again, this voice told him that it was time to get up. It was time.

Shortly after, Jasper made himself go to the GP to get help for his migraines. This is where our GP in the Hawaiian shirt makes his first appearance. Jasper doesn't recall much of that initial appointment but we can surmise that the GP suspected more was going on for him than migraines, because he was referred for a psychiatric assessment at a local mental health day hospital.

It was not, it turned out, an especially therapeutic introduction to mental health services. 'At that time I had no idea that there was this whole industry, this whole area of healthcare that's built around looking at somebody's experience as a disease. And intuitively, even back then, that didn't feel right.'

I've said that Jasper has a tendency to see the best in everyone. In truth, he struggles to find much that's good to say about the 'steroidal goliath of a mental health nurse' who first assessed him. Jasper recalls clinical, invasive and disconnected questions. He recalls his own paranoia, keeping his answers clipped, saying as little as he could get away with. He wanted to say that he was confused but was afraid to appear vulnerable. He never talked about the cameras that he could see in the corners of the rooms, his belief that he was always being watched. Or his more fleeting beliefs that he was Jim Morrison or God or undercover. He never talked about the time at university when he believed he could change a lecturer's argument simply by staring at him.

But whatever he did or did not say in that assessment resulted in a letter to his GP with its standard queries of psychosis and paranoia.

A week or so later he was back in the GP's consulting room and they were looking through the letter together. The GP read through it with him, then said, 'Oh, we don't really need that, do we?' He placed it to one side. It never made its way into Jasper's notes.

'He was an awesome GP,' Jasper says. 'Looking back, I'd say that maybe he'd experienced some mental health problems of his own and he just didn't want me to get sucked into that system.'

Another day, another story.

Jasper was referred back to the mental health day hospital for a few outpatient appointments. He was seen each week by a community mental health nurse who today he describes as his first nursing role model.

I ask him what they talked about.

'I have a vague recollection of unpacking this idea of paranoia with him. But I don't remember the content so much as a strong feeling of comfort, of feeling safe, feeling all right to talk to him. I didn't feel that I needed to talk about anything, but equally I felt that I could if I wanted to.'

Jasper also saw another nurse who specialised in psychotherapy. 'We spent a lot of time sitting in silence,' he recalls. 'It sounds bizarre. But it did me good because I was able to think through things in the presence of somebody else, without actually needing to say anything.'

The efficacy of psychotherapies for the treatment of psychosis is one hotly debated subject. I've talked a lot in this book about the ideological rift between those who are profoundly critical of the biomedical view of serious mental distress and those who seek to defend it. Seldom is this rift in sharper relief than when the subject of psychological therapies is on the table.

Jasper offers his take, which is based on his own published and ongoing research looking at some of the most complex patients in the country.

'CBT for psychosis isn't a panacea,' he begins. 'But it undoubtedly helps. And the mistake with comparing it to medication is that they do different things. CBT isn't a quasi-neuroleptic, and if you simply test for its effect in reducing psychotic symptoms – which is what the drugs are ultimately tested for – then you're not investigating what CBT actually does.'

And what does it do?

'So essentially the symptom profile of an individual may not change at all. CBT for psychosis doesn't necessarily get rid of the symptoms. And actually, sometimes they're just as prevalent in terms of frequency too. What changes, though, is the person's relationship with them. If they hear hostile voices then they aren't as distressed by them. They are more empowered over them. And that's a massive thing. Imagine if you're getting bullied at school, in the playground, and you feel awful about that and everything else. But I can help you to think of that bully in a completely different way. As somebody who can't hurt you, can't change your life, can't have this negative influence. The bully is still there. They're still going to do the same things, but you're not as bothered. You're better defended. That's what CBT does. So its usefulness depends which lens you're looking through. If you look at it from a traditional medical perspective, which prioritises amelioration of symptoms – a standard it frequently falls short of itself – then yes, it's ineffective. But if you look at it in terms of reducing depression, increasing quality of life, changing somebody's relationship with their experiences, then it's really effective.'

So that's Jasper's view. I'm inclined to afford it quite a bit of weight, not least because it has been forged at the sharpest end of psychiatry and is based on working with extremely distressed and unwell people.

Jasper's transition from someone whose life was being ruined by the voices in his head to a senior nurse who specialises in helping other voice hearers has clearly been a significant journey for him.

'I think one of the reasons for my going into psychiatric nursing was because I wanted to understand what was behind my assessor asking those questions,' he says. 'So becoming a nurse was almost a way to understand the system, to begin to see whether I trusted the system, to see whether I got it. Because the confusion I felt in that first assessment was just so great.'

Like myself and many other nurses, Jasper has worked in several settings; a career that for him has been largely mapped onto areas that have been most resistant to change. Forensic services are often perceived as the last stronghold for a staunchly biomedical approach. Certainly ten years ago, when Jasper first mooted the idea of a patient-led hearing voices support group,* it was something of a tumbleweed moment. *We don't do that kind of thing here.* It would be another seven years before it was established properly. More recently, the group has won awards for innovation. 'The group aims for people to feel more empowered and less isolated in relation to their voices,' Jasper says. 'That means they are less likely to act on those voices, particularly the ones which tell them to harm themselves or other people.'

---

* An idea inspired by the Hearing Voices Network (HVN), a national organisation of self-help groups run by and for people who hear voices. Though not overtly anti-psychiatry in its literature, HVN is certainly critical of many aspects of traditional psychiatry, and seeks to place greater emphasis on the content (rather than simply the presence) of voices, while accepting the explanations of each individual voice hearer with regard to the causes and meaning of their experience.

After clearing it with the group and the specialist service, Jasper invites me to attend one of their meetings.

———

I'll tell you about the group but first I want you to spend a moment trying to remember the the last time that you hallucinated.

Maybe it was when you read that last sentence – if your brain helpfully removed the extra 'the' between the words 'remember' and 'last'. Or maybe it was that time you felt your phone buzz in your pocket or heard it chime, only to take it out and realise there was no message waiting.

I imagine that many readers of this book will have personal experience of the more pronounced kind of hallucinations, as described to me by Jasper and others. But for readers who do not identify with such experiences, now seems a good moment to acknowledge that we do still hallucinate. Moreover, some of the most interesting and groundbreaking work in the study of hallucinations and voice hearing suggests that not only does everyone hallucinate but that we do so frequently.

'Most perception is controlled hallucination,' explains Dr Philip Corlett of the Yale School of Medicine. He's widely acknowledged to be leading the march on the neuroscience of hallucinations. 'There's a common misunderstanding of perception,' he continues, 'which is that we're bumbling around in the world and passively receiving information through our senses, rather like we're a video camera. In fact, it turns out – and we've known this for a long time – that perception is a much more synthetic or creative process. The brain is generative, it's constantly producing predictions about what is going to happen next based on our previous experiences. What we think we see and hear is not only formed from the information coming in through our senses, but also from this generative, predictive process.'

One plain example of this is how the brain fills in the gaps that we would otherwise experience in our field of vision. At the point where the optic nerve joins the back of the retina there are none of the rod and cone cells that perceive light. This results in a blind spot. As you read this book, there are parts of your wider visual field that you are not *seeing* with your eyes at all. Rather, they're being generated based entirely on what your brain *expects* to be there. If we define hallucinations as perceptions without external stimuli (and it's hard to know how else we might define them) then that's a very helpful little hallucination playing out for you right at this moment.

It doesn't stop there. The brain must frequently generate information, which we perceive as having arrived from our senses, in order to keep us safe.

Dr Corlett gives an example much like the one we encountered earlier in this book, when thinking about delusions. Imagine you're walking alone down a dark alleyway late at night. You're feeling on edge, maybe even afraid. If you hear an ambiguous background noise in such a scenario your brain may resolve this – at least momentarily – as being footsteps following you. 'It's a very efficient solution to the problem of perception being under-determined,' he says. 'Where uncertainty is high, it can be useful to fill in the details based on a set of predictions. It's conceivable that filling in uncertainty with a threatening explanation is helpful to us insofar as it's better to have a false alarm than miss an important signal that could be disastrous for our survival. Perhaps schizophrenia and psychosis are the price that we pay for using this sort of strategy. Being able to hallucinate might be very helpful, but not if you do it too much.'

That explanation may make sense in the context of a misinterpreted sound or an unexpected movement in the shadows. But that feels entirely different to the experience of hearing voices that speak in whole sentences.

'So one way of understanding the neuroanatomy of perception and cognition is that there is a *hierarchy of processing* that becomes increasingly abstract the further away it is from the initial sensation,' Dr Corlett tells me.

This is a little bit complicated (to me, anyway) but essentially we know that within each of our sensory systems – sight, hearing, smell and so on – there are many *layers* of activity going on within the brain. In the visual system, for instance, as we move through these layers different cells will code for particular visual properties: flashes of light become edges that become objects that become fully filled-in visual perceptions. That's the hierarchy of processing at work.

'Then things get especially interesting around a part of the brain called the lateral occipital complex,' Dr Corlett continues. 'This sits right at the top of this visual hierarchy. Here, things become *cognitive*. To help you interpret a visual sensation, information is brought in from other senses, lots of other senses, including your own sense of yourself. This, for me, is where meaning lives.'

Crucially, the movement of information in this hierarchy is not one-way. It doesn't all flow upwards from our sensory apparatus towards cognition, but rather it moves freely in both directions, with the higher regions of the brain sending their predictions downwards.

We might then conceive of more complex hallucinations (such as voices that speak in complete sentences or terrifying visions that no one else can see) as the result of an imbalance in this system, wherein those higher cognitive processes (drawing upon our pre-existing knowledge of the world and our place within it) have an exaggerated influence on the more basic perceptual processes beneath them (the ones that are just busy trying to turn light into shapes, and so on). The theory goes that if this imbalance becomes too exaggerated and those higher processes begin to exert too much influence then we will *literally* see and hear the things that we're thinking about – thoughts that may well be driven by our most pressing needs or worst fears.

It's a credible theory and one that may go some way towards bridging the void between the biological and the trauma-informed explanations of psychosis.

How so?

Well, as Philip Corlett explains, our beliefs and our perceptual conclusions are likely to be very, very sensitive to the degree of perceived uncertainty in the world around us. 'When perceptual uncertainty is higher,' he offers, 'when there's more noise in the system, we must rely more on our prior beliefs in order to reconcile that uncertainty. Because the bottom line for the application of all of these models to psychosis, and more broadly to anxiety and PTSD, is that as organisms we really hate any kind of uncertainty about what's going to happen to us and will do anything we can – including experience horrifying symptoms – in order to reconcile that uncertainty. Hallucinations and delusions are stories that we tell ourselves in order that we can make better predictions about what's going to happen to us next.'

He's keen to stress that life trauma is not a prerequisite of hallucinations but that this theory is nonetheless aligned to the observed higher rates of psychosis in people who have suffered trauma. 'If your model of the world through development is that you can't even rely on your parents to take care of you,' he offers by way of example, 'then that's a shortcut to massive amounts of uncertainty about other individuals and situations.'

Of course, if this 'predictive processing' theory of hallucinations is correct then we would expect people to hallucinate less often in times of lower stress and greater certainty. And there's no doubt that this is a message we hear time and again from voice hearers.

'If you can engage in behaviours that help you to reduce uncertainty, that often seems to help,' reflects Dr Corlett. 'We're often told by voice hearers that listening to music helps. It's not just that you're distracted by some other auditory stimulus, but that the auditory stimulus is providing a structure that leaves less room for uncertainty to influence what's being perceived. Being in a calm, predictable environment that mitigates uncertainty – and so reduces the need to rely on prior beliefs to reconcile that uncertainty – is likely to help people hear voices less frequently. The same account could be extended to delusions, too.'[1]

———

It's evening when Jasper and I arrive at the hospital and, looking up through the darkness at the perimeter fence, I note the same perceptible tightening in my chest that I felt some twenty years ago when I stepped onto a non-secure psychiatric ward for the very first time.

Once we're inside the bright, open foyer area, however, I'm relieved to feel that I'm very much in a hospital and not a prison – just a hospital with notably enhanced security.

Jasper leads me along echoey corridors, through a succession of locked doors. I become very conscious of the fact that he has keys but as a visitor I do not. I don't feel afraid, as such, but there's no doubt that my senses feel heightened, hyper-alert. It crosses my mind that this must certainly be the case for the patients, too.

The Hearing Voices Support Group takes place in a well-lit and airy room. We wait for the patients to be brought over from their respective wards, and one by one they're introduced to me. They knew I was coming, of course. In fact, long before I had any contact with Jasper a few of them had read my novel as part of a hospital reading group, so I'm afforded the flattering status of a visiting author. Such ceremony doesn't last long. I'm relieved when one of the men breaks the ice by telling me a joke about a patient, a psychiatrist, a roll of cling film and a pair of testicles. I probably shouldn't repeat it. But it's a good 'un.

Once we're all seated around the table – Jasper, myself, another nurse and about eight patients – the session begins. We go around the table with everyone introducing themselves and saying a few words about how their voices have been affecting them since the last meeting. We get to Jasper and he does exactly the same. Here's the thing: voices remain a part of Jasper's life to this day.

It was a huge moment, the first time he volunteered to the group about his own personal experience. They had been meeting every couple of months for about two years before he did so, and he had agonised over the decision.

What personal information nurses should or shouldn't disclose to their patients is frequently debated in our professional community and, I suspect, nowhere more so than in the field of forensic mental health. 'We're supposed to be there for them, not the other way round,' Jasper had said to me, when we first talked about this. 'It's not their responsibility to help me.'

At the same time, while facilitating the group for those first two years he hadn't been able to shake the feeling that sharing his experience was what he was supposed to do; that it would be helpful for his patients. After much soul-searching over many months, and after gaining the appropriate permissions, he made the decision to disclose.

'We were going round the table, checking in,' he explained, 'and it got to me. And I said, "I feel like I've been a slight fraud with you guys." Then I told them. I told them my history. Then I gave an example of voices I'd heard in the past few weeks, exactly as they do. I just put it there on the table, and then there was this silence and I thought: Oh God, there's no turning back.'

However vulnerable and fearful Jasper felt in those first few minutes, his disclosure proved to be absolutely the right call.

'In that moment, it stopped being us and them. It stopped being a keyholder and non-keyholders. It was just a group of voice hearers talking about our experiences, talking about what works for us, what doesn't work for us . . .'

At the end of the sessions, a standard ritual plays out, where the men say their goodbyes to each other before being taken back to their respective locked wards. It's all fist bumps and man hugs. Needless to say, in a forensic setting, the nurses don't join in with that.

On that day, one of the lads put a firm hand on Jasper's shoulder and hugged him, too. Then they all did. As Jasper tells me this, it's clear that he remains deeply moved by the experience. 'The funny thing is,' he adds, 'they each kept just enough of a gap between us so as not to touch my key belt and infringe any security protocols. They know I go home at the end of a shift. I can see my family whenever I want. I can go to the shops. My day isn't ordered by security protocols. I've got all of these luxuries. By the nature of it, there are some distressed, vulnerable, violent people who really believe they are in danger and so will defend themselves. Or they're working through some nasty, nasty stuff. And of course a part of my mind is always on security because that's the context in which I work. I worry about the group members, say if one of them is dipping. I'll worry about where that may or may not take him. And I'm one of the people who might need to restrain that individual. I'm a restrainer, I'm a custodian, I'm a keyholder, I'm a nurse. They all know that. But actually, when I'm in the group, I'm just a part of that group.'

When arranging to attend the group myself I had to offer some assurances. I said that I wouldn't name the hospital and that I wouldn't report specific details of anything that was disclosed by any of the men. I wouldn't bring a pen in and I wouldn't take a narrative out.

So, once again, we are left with the feelings. Here's the best way I can describe the feelings that I detected in that room.

Imagine, once more, that you're walking down that dark alley we've been talking about. You hear the sudden noise. It's footsteps. Only this time, it doesn't resolve itself to be rustling leaves by virtue of you listening more attentively. It remains footsteps. It's always footsteps. Something is always following you. Always wanting to harm you. And it's caught you before, whatever this thing is, and when it did, when that happened, it was too terrifying to contemplate. Now imagine you look to your left, and there's a friend walking beside you. Your friend can hear the footsteps behind you, too. And to your right is another friend, and another, and another.

You're not alone at all. There's a whole gang of you. You're all walking this dark alley together. It's longer than you thought. It's darker than you feared. But you're doing it, and come to think of it, when you're all together like this – your own footsteps sound the loudest.

That was the feeling in the room.

That's what I took away.

Leaving the Heartland

THIS IS WHERE WE PART COMPANY.

It's been quite a journey, hasn't it? It certainly has been for me. At the start of this book I mentioned how difficult I once found it to write a novel. I've now discovered that writing this kind of book is not without its challenges either.

The people we've met and spent time with are as real as you and me. They welcomed me into their lives and allowed me to share their stories. That's felt like a pretty major responsibility. It's also opened my eyes to things that even as a mental health nurse I'd never fully appreciated. In my nursing role, I was part of a psychiatric system that I've been forced to re-evaluate, as we've explored in these pages exactly what it means to be medically assessed, diagnosed and treated for our thoughts, feelings and behaviours.

We've seen that the most distressing personal experiences – those that lead to the diagnosis of mental disorders – are as likely to be shaped by our relationships and the pressures of our environment as they are by any abnormalities in our biology, and that sometimes what needs 'fixing' mightn't reside within the individual at all. We've seen that this often gets overlooked by well-meaning anti-stigma campaigns, and have considered why this could be in the interests of governments and powerful institutions.

By examining how doctors arrive at psychiatric diagnoses we have come to realise that the science behind this is fundamentally flawed.

We've learnt how genes can increase our susceptibility to certain kinds of suffering. But we've also seen that it would be wrong to conclude that such genetic variation is necessarily a bad thing.

We've seen how foetal or early-life events can change the structure of our brain in ways that have far-reaching consequences for our mental wellbeing, while acknowledging that the vast majority of 'mental disorders' cannot be observed on the physical matter of the brain.

We have discovered that strange experiences such as hallucinations and delusions may be nothing more than extensions of entirely healthy thinking strategies designed to keep us safe, and how changing our relationship with these experiences can go a long way towards reducing the distress that they cause.

By taking a close look at psychiatric medication we've revealed that nobody fully understands how these chemicals work. We have seen both the good and the harm caused by antipsychotic drugs, and have shone a light on cracks in the evidence behind current prescribing practices.

We have witnessed mental health services supporting people and we've witnessed them failing people.

Above all, we have found that nothing in the world of mental health is uncontroversial. Almost everything remains in dispute. Yet by spending time with Amit, Molly, James, Clare and Joe, Kate and Brigid, and Jasper, I believe we have arrived at one clear and indisputable truth. It is that when we talk about mental illness, we are talking about people.

Our journey has only taken us so far. I'm mindful of how much there is that we haven't seen. Earlier in this book, I described schizophrenia as the 'heartland of psychiatry'; a place from which we could explore – and hopefully come to better understand – contested notions of mental health and illness.

The heartland, it turns out, is a mountainous region with many false peaks. The view from here may well be more expansive than it was from where we began but we're still nowhere near the summit.

And at the risk of stretching the metaphor, we've only taken the Western ascent, focusing on Western experiences, ideas and treatments. There are other routes that we could have taken, and we might be surprised at how different the view looks from those.

In 1979, the World Health Organisation (WHO) announced the findings of a five-year study which showed that people with a diagnosis of schizophrenia in developing countries fared better than those living in wealthy, industrialised nations. That was a hard pill to swallow (at least it was for those in the countries with the best pills), and yet a huge follow-up study, conducted across ten countries over two years, confirmed the findings. Patients living in poorer nations enjoyed higher levels of social functioning and longer periods of remission than those living in nations with the most advanced medical resources and technologies.[1]

Nobody has been able to definitively explain the reasons for this. There is still much left to explore.

But I do believe we've covered some significant ground. In the first chapter I asked you to say 'schizophrenia' out loud. To say it loud enough that you would be heard. To repeat it, feel the shape of it, stay with it. I asked you to reflect upon what thoughts and feelings this word arrived with.

If you do that again now, I wonder if some of your thoughts and feelings will have changed?

Mine have.

We've just heard the story of a keyholder. But we're all keyholders of sorts, aren't we? We make decisions about people based on ideas and orthodoxies that we may never once have questioned. We place people in the corners of our minds, locking them away there. Sometimes we do the same to ourselves.

I hope that this book has been able to unlock a few such doors. To push them open, though, requires more than I can do here. It involves many people having many more conversations.

My hope now is that you – *yes, you!* – will take the conversation that we've started here and continue it with others.

It's about all of us.

By talking and listening carefully we can push those doors wide open. I wonder what else we'll find?

It's a beginning.

Acknowledgements

At the heart of this book are the people who shared their stories with me. Some of those stories appear in these pages; others do not but were nonetheless invaluable in shaping my knowledge and understanding. Given that some of the contributors asked to have their names changed (and that it would feel odd to include pseudonyms in these acknowledgements) I'll simply say that you each know who you are and that I'm so very grateful to you.

Thank you also to the mental health clinicians, academics and other experts who corresponded with me. Although in the Venn diagram of your ideas there isn't always much overlap, what you all so clearly have in common is the desire to better understand what it means to be human and to help those who are suffering. You are: Wendy Burn, Anne Cooke, Philip Corlett, Megan Cowles, Anthony David, Jacqui Dillon, Daniel Freeman, Suzi Gage, Joel Gold, Sameer Jauhar, Doreen Joseph, Alex Langford, Simon McCarthy-Jones, Joanna Moncrieff, Martha Parker, Vanessa Pinfold, John Read, Graham Thornicroft, André Tomlin, Agata Vitale and Jessica Woolley.

A very special thank-you to the psychologists Lucy Johnstone and John McGowan, and to the psychiatrists Robin Murray and James Walters. You each went above and beyond.

Thank you to my editor Lou Joyner, whose intelligence, sensitivity and compassion have been a guiding light throughout this endeavour. Also to Maria Garbutt-Lucero, John Grindrod, Libby Marshall, Ruth O'Loughlin, Anne Owen, Sophie Portas, David Woodhouse and the rest of the team at Faber, and to my copy editor Eleanor Rees.

Thank you, as ever, to my brilliant agent Sophie Lambert at C&W.

I'm grateful to my parents, who take such an interest in my writing, and to my children, who take such an interest in interrupting it. Both are useful in their own ways. Thank you also to my mother-in-law, Sue Parker, whose help looking after the children has afforded me so much more time to write.

Other dear friends and companions along the way have been Tanya Atapattu, Phil Bambridge, Sarah Bambridge, Mark Barron, Kate Button, Rosy Carrick, Ben and Zia Clarke, Chelsey Flood, Craig Flowers, Jamie Harrison, Kev Hawkins, Andy Marshall, Molly Naylor, Ruth Sayers and Polly Weston.

Finally, Emily Parker. I could easily include you in the list of mental health experts. But then I'd have nobody to put in this final list of best friend, wife and hero.

Notes

The Language of Madness

1 For an interesting debate about what is the most appropriate collective noun to describe those of us who use mental health services, read: Christmas, David M. B., and Sweeney, Angela, 'Service User, Patient, Survivor or Client . . . Has the Time Come to Return to "Patient"?', *British Journal of Psychiatry* 209 (2016), 9–13.

2 Filer, N., *The Shock of the Fall* (HarperCollins, 2013), 233.

3 Goodwin, G. M., and Geddes, J. R., 'What Is the Heartland of Psychiatry?', *British Journal of Psychiatry* 191 (2007), 189–91.

4 'Psychiatrists and Psychologists Pledge to End "Bitter" Adversarial Dynamic', *Mental Health Today*, 27 November 2018. https://www.mentalhealthtoday.co.uk/news/mental-health-profession/psychiatrists-and-psychologists-pledges-to-end-bitter-adversarial-dynamic

5 In describing my first day of working on a psychiatric ward I have quoted from my own BBC Radio 4 documentary, *The Mind in the Media*. https://www.bbc.co.uk/programmes/b08hl265

6 Elyn Saks's TED talk is 'A Tale of Mental Illness – from the Inside', www.ted.com/talks/elyn_saks_seeing_mental_illness/ She also describes her experiences in extraordinarily vivid detail in her memoir, *The Centre Cannot Hold* (Hachette, 2007).

7 For a heartbreakingly poetic take on the 'one in a hundred' statistic, read: *Uninvited Guest* by Jenny Robertson (Triangle, 1997).

8 'Mimsy Were the Borogoves', *Detective Comics* 1, no. 789 (2003).

The Journalist

1 This conversation formed part of my BBC Radio 4 documentary *The Mind in the Media*. https://www.bbc.co.uk/programmes/b08hl265

Insight

1   From the 2018 lecture 'Knowing Me, Knowing You: Insight in
    Psychiatry and Medicine' by Anthony S. David (part of The King's
    Lectures at King's College London and now available on YouTube).

2   This conversation with Ann Dines is recorded in Hugh W. Diamond's
    1856 paper 'On the Application of Photography to the Physiognomic
    and Mental Phenomena of Insanity', which has been reproduced
    along with a remarkable collection of his photographic plates in *The
    Face of Madness: Hugh W. Diamond and the Origin of Psychiatric
    Photography*, edited by Sander L. Gilman (EPBM, 1976).

3   Steinman, M. A., Shlipak, M. G., and McPhee, S. J., 'Of Principles and
    Pens: Attitudes and Practices of Medicine Housestaff toward
    Pharmaceutical Industry Promotions', *American Journal of Medicine*
    110:7 (2001), 551–7. PMID: 11347622

4   Gregory Zilboorg quote cited in Reddy, M. S., 'Insight and Psychosis',
    Indian Journal of Psychological Medicine 37:3 (2015), 257–60.
    doi:10.4103/0253-7176.162909

5   The quotations from Robin Murray throughout this book are from
    my interview with him in February 2018.

6   Aubrey Lewis quote cited in David, A. S., 'Insight and Psychosis', *British
    Journal of Psychiatry* 156 (1990), 798–808. For a further discussion of
    Lewis's insights on insight (complete with a nod to Rabbie Burns) read:
    David, A. S., '"To See Oursels as Others See Us." Aubrey Lewis's Insight',
    British Journal of Psychiatry 174 (1999), 210–16.

7   Laing, R. D., *The Politics of Experience* (Penguin Books, 1990), 115.

8   Bedford, N. J., et al., 'Self-evaluation in Schizophrenia: an fMRI Study
    with Implications for the Understanding of Insight', *BMC Psychiatry*
    12 (2012), 106. http://www.biomedcentral.com/1471-244X/12/106

9   Button, Katherine S., et al., 'Power Failure: Why Small Sample Size
    Undermines the Reliability of Neuroscience', *Nature Reviews
    Neuroscience* 14 (2013), 365–76. doi:10.1038/nrn3475

10 Colorado State University, 'Brain Images Make Cognitive Research
    More Believable', *ScienceDaily*, 8 October 2007. www.sciencedaily.com/
    releases/2007/10/071002151837.htm

11 Kupfer, D., 'Chair of DSM-5 Task Force Discusses Future of Mental
    Health Research', News release, American Psychiatric Association,
    3 May 2013.

12 The Hippocrates quote appears in *The Genuine Works of Hippocrates*, translated by F. Adams (W. Wood, 1886), vol. 2, 344–5.

13 University of California – Berkeley, 'Physicists, Engineers to Build Next-generation MRI Brain Scanner', 6 October 2017. https://phys.org/news/2017-10-physicists-next-generation-mri-brain-scanner.html

14 As discussed in the *Radiolab* episode 'Blame': https://www.wnycstudios.org/story/317421-blame

15 Lysaker, Paul H., et al., 'Toward Understanding the Insight Paradox: Internalized Stigma Moderates the Association Between Insight and Social Functioning, Hope, and Self-esteem among People with Schizophrenia Spectrum Disorders', *Schizophrenia Bulletin* 33: 1 (2007), 192–9. doi:10.1093/schbul/sbl016

Stigma and Discrimination

1 This quotation, along with my reflections on how this story made me feel, formed part of the BBC Radio 4 documentary *The Mind in the Media*. https://www.bbc.co.uk/programmes/b08hl265

2 Brekke, J. S., Prindle, C., Bae, S. W., and Long, J. D., 'Risks for Individuals with Schizophrenia Who Are Living in the Community', *Psychiatric Services* 52 (2001), 1358–66. doi: 10.1176/appi.ps.52.10.1358

3 You can find out more about Recovery in the Bin at their website: https://recoveryinthebin.org/

4 For a readable discussion of these figures, see the Living With Schizophrenia website: https://www.livingwithschizophreniauk.org/information-sheets/can-you-recover-from-schizophrenia/. For a more robust meta-analysis on recovery look at: Jääskeläinen, E., Juola, P., Hirvonen, N., McGrath, J. J., Saha, S., Isohanni, M., Veijola, J., and Miettunen, J., 'A Systematic Review and Meta-Analysis of Recovery in Schizophrenia', *Schizophrenia Bulletin* 39:6 (2013), 1296–1306. https://doi.org/10.1093/schbul/sbs130

5 This quotation is from Graham Thornicroft's book *Shunned: Discrimination against People with Mental Illness* (OUP, 2006). The subsequent quotations are from my own interview with him in February 2017.

6 Statistic from 'Thriving at Work: a Review of Mental Health and Employers', commissioned by the UK government and published in 2017.

7 This full essay by Anne Cooke and Dave Harper can be found at http://discursiveoftunbridgewells.blogspot.co.uk/2013/05/when-ads-dont-work.html

8 Quote from: https://www.bbc.co.uk/mediacentre/latestnews/2016/in-the-mind

9 A copy of the full letter can be found at: http://peterkinderman.blogspot.co.uk/2016/02/open-letter-about-bbc-coverage-of.html?m=1

10 The quotations from Dr Lucy Johnstone throughout this book are taken from my interview with her in February 2018.

11 Time to Change statistics from: http://www.time-to-change.org.uk/about-us/our-impact

12 Henderson, C., Robinson, E., Evans-Lacko, S., Corker, E., Rebollo-Mesa, I., Rose, D., and Thornicroft, G., 'Public Knowledge, Attitudes, Social Distance and Reported Contact regarding People with Mental Illness 2009–2015', *Acta Psychiatrica Scandinavica* 134 (suppl. 446) (2016), 23–33.

13 Kvaal, E. P., Gottdiener, W. H., and Haslam, N., 'Biogenetic Explanations and Stigma: A Meta-analytic Review of Associations among Laypeople', *Social Science and Medicine* 96 (2013), 95–103; Angermeyer, M. C., Holzinger, A., Carta, M. G., and Schomerus, G., 'Biogenetic Explanations and Public Acceptance of Mental Illness: Systematic Review of Population Studies', *British Journal of Psychiatry* 199 (2011), 367–72.

14 This argument is made by Joanna Moncrieff in *A Straight Talking Introduction to Psychiatric Drugs* (PCCS Books, 2009). This is one of a series of *Straight Talking Introductions to Mental Health Problems* edited by Richard Bentall and Pete Sanders. I recommend them as an accessible way into critical thinking about psychiatry and mental health. We'll meet Dr Moncrieff in person later in this book.

15 The full post, which includes more clinical details than I've quoted here, can be found at https://psychiatrysho.wordpress.com/2015/06/10/is-depression-really-like-diabetes-yes-but-maybe-not-how-you-imagined/

Diagnosis

1 For an interesting discussion on this, and on diagnostic reliability
   more broadly, read: Aboraya, A., Rankin, E., France, C., El-Missiry,
   A., and John, C., 'The Reliability of Psychiatric Diagnosis Revisited:
   The Clinician's Guide to Improve the Reliability of Psychiatric
   Diagnosis', *Psychiatry (Edgmont)* 3:1 (2006), 41–50.

2 Kendell, R. E., Cooper, J. E., Gourlay, A. J., Copeland, J. R. M., Sharpe,
   L., and Gurland, B. J., 'Diagnostic Criteria of American and British
   Psychiatrists', *Archives of General Psychiatry* 25:2 (1971), 123–30.
   doi:10.1001/archpsyc.1971.01750140027006

3 To hear audio footage of David Rosenhan discussing this, you might
   like to listen to my own BBC Radio 4 documentary: *The Mind in the
   Media*. https://www.bbc.co.uk/programmes/b08hl265

4 From Rosenhan, D. L., 'On Being Sane in Insane Places', *Science*,
   19 January 1973, 250–8.

5 American Psychiatric Association, *Diagnostic and Statistical Manual
   of Mental Disorders*, 2nd edn (1968), 40

6 American Psychiatric Association, *Diagnostic and Statistical Manual
   of Mental Disorders*, 3rd edn (1980), 213–15.

7 My summaries of Lucy Johnstone's arguments through the remainder
   of this chapter are taken from our interview in 2018 and also from
   Johnstone, Lucy, *A Straight Talking Introduction to Psychiatric
   Diagnosis* (PCCS Books, 2014).

8 Insel, Thomas, 'Transforming Diagnosis', National Institute of Mental
   Health (2013). https://www.nimh.nih.gov/about/directors/thomas-
   insel/blog/2013/transforming-diagnosis.shtml

9 Kupfer, D., 'Chair of DSM-5 Task Force Discusses Future of Mental
   Health Research', News release, American Psychiatric Association,
   3 May 2013.

10 For more on the political struggles behind the DSM and a more
   rigorous history of it in general, I recommend: Blashfield, Roger K.,
   Keeley, Jared W., Flanagan, Elizabeth H., and Miles, Shannon R., 'The
   Cycle of Classification: DSM-I through DSM-5', *Annual Review of
   Clinical Psychology* 10:1 (2014), 25–51.

11 Daniel Carlat's recollection of this interview with Robert Spitzer can
   be found at: https://www.mdedge.com/psychiatry/article/105698/
   dr-robert-spitzer-personal-tribute. I discovered the anecdote in

Cracked: Why Psychiatry is Doing More Harm Than Good by James
Davies (Icon Books, 2013).

12   Hyman is quoted in 'Psychiatry's Guide Is Out of Touch With
Science, Experts Say', *New York Times*, 6 May 2013

13   Quoted from Sami Timimi, 'No More Psychiatric Labels', *Asylum*,
May 2012: http://asylummagazine.org/2012/05/no-more-psychiatric-
labels/

14   Murray, R., 'Mistakes I Have Made in My Research Career',
Schizophrenia Bulletin 43:2 (2017), 253–6.

The Mother

1   A version of Clare's letter to Joe has been published in the *Guardian*
newspaper: 'A letter to . . . my late son, who had schizophrenia', 5
February 2011. https://www.theguardian.com/lifeandstyle/2011/
feb/05/letter-to-my-late-son-who-had-schizophrenia

Causes

1   As revealed by Rethink: https://www.rethink.org/media/1178709/
plus_twenty_report.pdf

2   Mattila, T., Koeter, M., Wohlfarth, T., Storosum, J., van den Brink, W.,
de Haan, L., Derks, E., Leufkens, H., and Denys, D., 'Impact of DSM-
5 Changes on the Diagnosis and Acute Treatment of Schizophrenia',
Schizophrenia Bulletin 41: 3 (1 May 2015), 637–43. doi.org/10.1093/
schbul/sbu172

3   Evidence of this is found across the literature. For a readable
summary and discussion of some of the most prominent (though
occasionally contentious) psycho-social research see: Cooke, A. (ed.),
Understanding Psychosis and Schizophrenia (British Psychological
Society, 2014).

4   Hughes, K., et al., 'The Effect of Multiple Adverse Childhood
Experiences on Health: A Systematic Review and Meta-analysis',
Lancet Public Health 2 (2017), e356–66. doi.org/10.1016/S2468-
2667(17)30118-4

5   Varese, F., Smeets, F., Drukker, M., Lieverse, R., Lataster, T.,

Viechtbauer, W., Read, J., van Os, J., and Bentall, R. P., 'Childhood Adversities Increase the Risk of Psychosis: A Meta-analysis of Patient-Control, Prospective- and Cross-sectional Cohort Studies', *Schizophrenia Bulletin* 38:4 (2012), 661–71. doi.org/10.1093/schbul/sbs050

6   See NSPCC website: https://www.nspcc.org.uk/preventing-abuse/child-abuse-and-neglect/child-sexual-abuse/sexual-abuse-facts-statistics/

7   Read, J., et al., 'Child Maltreatment and Psychosis: A Return to a Genuinely Integrated Bio-psycho-social Model', *Clinical Schizophrenia and Related Psychoses* 2:3 (2008), 235–54.

8   Morgan, C., et al., 'Parental Separation, Loss and Psychosis in Different Ethnic Groups: A Case-control Study', *Psychological Medicine* 37:4 (2007), 495–503. doi:10.1017/S0033291706009330

9   My summary of Simon McCarthy-Jones's argument is taken from his excellent book, *Can't You Hear Them? The Science and Significance of Hearing Voices* (Jessica Kingsley, 2017), 44.

10 Scotland is stealing a march on this, not only in mental healthcare but across its public-sector workforce. NHS Education for Scotland has even produced a film about it, called 'Opening Doors: Trauma Informed Practice for the Workforce'. You can find it here: https://vimeo.com/274703693

11 Read, J., Harper, D., Tucker, I., and Kennedy, A., 'Do Adult Mental Health Services Identify Child Abuse and Neglect? A Systematic Review', *International Journal of Mental Health Nursing* 27 (2018), 7–19. doi:10.1111/inm.12369

12 Harrington, A., 'The Fall of the Schizophrenogenic Mother', *Lancet* 379:9823 (2012), 1292–3.

13 John Read's arguments are taken from our correspondence and from his lecture 'The Psycho-social Causes of Distress and Madness: A Research Update', presented on 8 June 2018 at the University of East London. Also from Chapter 14 of *Models of Madness: Psychological, Social and Biological Approaches to Psychosis* (2nd edn, 2013), edited by John Read and Jacqui Dillon.

14 Wilkinson, R., and Pickett, K., 'Inequality and Mental Illness: Comment', *Lancet Psychiatry*, May 2017. https://www.equalitytrust.org.uk/inequality-and-mental-illness-comment-lancet-psychiatry-professors-wilkinson-and-pickett

15   Johnstone, L., and Boyle, M., with Cromby, J., Dillon, J., Harper, D.,
     Kinderman, P., Longden, E., Pilgrim, D., and Read, J., *The Power
     Threat Meaning Framework: Towards the identification of patterns in
     emotional distress, unusual experiences and troubled or troubling
     behaviour, as an alternative to functional psychiatric diagnosis* (British
     Psychological Society, 2018).

16   The quotations and references to Swaran Singh's arguments are taken
     from Singh, S. P., and Burns, T., 'Race and Mental Health: There Is
     More to Race than Racism', *British Medical Journal* 333:7569 (2006),
     648–51. doi:10.1136/bmj.38930.501516.BE, and from his appearance
     on the BBC *Horizon* documentary *Why Did I Go Mad?* You can listen
     to his interview on Soundcloud here: https://soundcloud.com/
     kidfinish-1/professor-swaran-singh-on-the-links-between-social-
     marginalisation-and-psychosis

17   Sundquist, K., Frank, G., and Sundquist, J., 'Urbanisation and
     Incidence of Psychosis and Depression: Follow-up Study of 4.4
     Million Women and Men in Sweden', *British Journal of Psychiatry*
     184:4 (2004), 293–8. doi:10.1192/bjp.184.4.293

18   Jongsma, H. E., Gayer-Anderson, C., Lasalvia, A., et al., 'Treated
     Incidence of Psychotic Disorders in the Multinational EU-GEI
     Study', *JAMA Psychiatry* 75:1 (2018), 36–46. doi:10.1001/
     jamapsychiatry.2017.3554

19   Di Forti, Marta, Marconi, Arianna, Carra, Elena, et al., 'Proportion of
     Patients in South London with First-episode Psychosis Attributable
     to Use of High Potency Cannabis: A Case-control Study', *Lancet
     Psychiatry* 2:3 (March 2015), 233–8.

20   Paul D. Morrison and Robin M. Murray, 'The Antipsychotic
     Landscape: Dopamine and Beyond', *Therapeutic Advancements in
     Psychopharmacology*, 23 January 2018.
     doi:10.1177/2045125317752915

21   *ibid*.

22   Suzi Gage's argument is taken from our correspondence in 2018 and
     from her *Guardian* newspaper article: 'So Smoking Skunk Causes
     Psychosis, But Milder Cannabis Doesn't?', 16 February 2015.

23   Schizophrenia Working Group of the Psychiatric Genomics
     Consortium, 'Biological Insights from 108 Schizophrenia-associated
     Genetic Loci', *Nature* 511 (2014), 421–7.

24   Lichtenstein, P., Yip, B. H., Björk, C., et al., 'Common Genetic

Determinants of Schizophrenia and Bipolar Disorder in Swedish Families: A Population-based Study', *Lancet* 373 (2009), 234–9.

25 Cross-Disorder Group of the Psychiatric Genomics Consortium, 'Genetic Relationship between Five Psychiatric Disorders Estimated from Genome-wide SNPs', *Nature Genetics* 45 (2013), 984–94.

26 Rees, E., Kirov, G., Sanders, A., Walters, J. T. R., et al., 'Evidence that Duplications of 22q11.2 Protect against Schizophrenia', *Molecular Psychiatry* 19 (2014), 37–40.

27 Here's the video: 'Where Everyone Wants to Be Your Friend', https://abcnews.go.com/2020/video/williams-syndrome-children-friend-health-disease-hospital-doctors-13817012

28 St Clair, D., Xu, M., Wang, P., et al., 'Rates of Adult Schizophrenia following Prenatal Exposure to the Chinese Famine of 1959–1961', *Journal of the American Medical Association* 294:5 (2005), 557–62. doi:10.1001/jama.294.5.557

29 For more information on neurodevelopmental theories of schizophrenia, see Haut, K. M., Schvarcz, A., Cannon, T. D., and Bearden, C. E., 'Neurodevelopmental Theories of Schizophrenia: Twenty-First Century Perspectives', in *Developmental Psychopathology*, ed. D. Cicchetti (2016). doi:10.1002/9781119125556.devpsy223

30 For a more detailed discussion of the 'synaptic pruning' hypothesis, see Boksa, P., 'Abnormal Synaptic Pruning in Schizophrenia: Urban Myth or Reality?', *Journal of Psychiatry and Neuroscience* 37:2 (2012), 75–7. http://doi.org/10.1503/jpn.120007

31 Read, J., et al., 'The Traumagenic Neurodevelopmental Model of Psychosis Revisited', *Neuropsychiatry* 4:1 (2014), 65–79.

32 The quotations from Joanna Moncrieff in this chapter and throughout the remainder of the book are from my interview with her in August 2018. She told me that she borrowed her description of schizophrenia as 'a way of being human' from the book *Schizophrenia: A Disease or Some Ways of Being Human?* by Alec Jenner et al. (Continuum, 1993). Moncrieff also writes about this in her blog at https://joannamoncrieff.com/2017/03/27/why-i-dont-like-the-idea-that-mental-disorder-is-a-disease/

33 Thomas Insel quoted in: https://www.wired.com/2017/05/star-neuroscientist-tom-insel-leaves-google-spawned-verily-startup/

Delusions

1 Knobloch-Westerwick, S., and Meng, J., 'Looking the Other Way: Selective Exposure to Attitude-consistent and Counter-attitudinal Political Information', *Communication Research* 36:3 (June 2009), 426–48.

2 American Psychiatric Association, *Diagnostic and Statistical Manual of Mental Disorders*, 5th edn (2013), 87.

3 This is an observation made in *Suspicious Minds: How Culture Shapes Madness* by Joel Gold and Ian Gold (Free Press, 2014). We'll meet Joel Gold later in the chapter.

4 The quotations from Daniel Freeman are taken from my interview with him in September 2018. For an academic review of his research, I recommend: Freeman, D., and Garety, P., 'Advances in Understanding and Treating Persecutory Delusions: A Review', *Social Psychiatry and Psychiatric Epidemiology* 49:8 (2014), 1179–89. doi. org/10.1007/s00127-014-0928-7

5 This cognitive bias is called the 'availability heuristic'. More on it here: Schwarz, N., Bless, H., Strack, F., Klumpp, G., Rittenauer-Schatka, H., and Simons, A., 'Ease of Retrieval as Information: Another Look at the Availability Heuristic', *Journal of Personality and Social Psychology* 61:2 (1991), 195–202. doi:10.1037/0022-3514.61.2.195

6 Freeman, D., Dunn, G., Startup, H., Pugh, K., Cordwell, J., Mander, H., et al., 'Effects of Cognitive Behaviour Therapy for Worry on Persecutory Delusions in Patients with Psychosis (WIT): a Parallel, Single-blind, Randomised Controlled Trial with a Mediation Analysis', *Lancet Psychiatry* 2 (2015), 305–13. doi: 10.1016/s2215-0366(15)00039-5

7 This quotation is from *Suspicious Minds: How Culture Shapes Madness* by Joel Gold and Ian Gold (Free Press, 2014), 228. The subsequent quotations from Joel Gold are taken from this work and from my interview with him in August 2018.

8 For more on dual-process accounts of reasoning, read: Evans, Jonathan St. B. T., 'In Two Minds: Dual-process Accounts of Reasoning', *Trends in Cognitive Sciences* 7:10 (2003), 454–9. doi. org/10.1016/j.tics.2003.08.012

9 Skodlar, B., et al., 'Psychopathology of Schizophrenia in Ljubljana (Slovenia) from 1881 to 2000: Changes in the Content of Delusions in Schizophrenia Patients Related to Various Sociopolitical, Technical

and Scientific Changes', *International Journal of Social Psychiatry* 54:2 (2008), 101–11. doi.org/10.1177/0020764007083875

10   The theory that delusions are an attempt to explain abnormal experiences such as hallucinations was first proposed by Brendan Maher in 1974. Much has been written about this since (including no shortage of criticism). Here's the original paper: Maher, B. A., 'Delusional Thinking and Perceptual Disorder', *Journal of Individual Psychology* 30 (1974), 98–113.

Chemical Treatment

1   The report, called 'Modernising the Mental Health Act: Increasing Choice, Reducing Compulsion: Final Report of the Independent Review of the Mental Health Act 1983' (December 2018) can be found at https://www.mentalhealthtoday.co.uk/media/32267/irmha1983_final-report.pdf

2   The quotation from Steve Gilbert is taken from an article in the *Independent*: 'Mental Health Act "Needs Major Reform" as Black Patients Four Times as Likely as Whites to Be Sectioned', 5 December 2018. https://www.independent.co.uk/news/health/mental-health-act-detained-sectioned-ethnic-minority-bme-report-nhs-a8669246.html

3   Swazey, J., *Chlorpromazine in Psychiatry* (Massachusetts Institute of Technology, 1974), 78.

4   Laborit, H., and Huguenard, P., 'L'Hibernation artificielle par moyens pharmacodynamiques et physiques' ['Artificial hibernation by physical and pharmacodynamic means'], *Presse Médicale* 59 (1951), 1329.

5   Anton-Stephens, D., 'Preliminary Observations on the Psychiatric Uses of Chlorpromazine (Largactil)', *Journal of Mental Science* 100 (1954), 543–57.

6   This account can be found in: Delay, J., and Deniker, P., '38 cas de psychoses traitées par la cure prolongée et continué de 4560 R.P.', *Comptes rendus du 50e Congrès des Médecins Aliénistes et Neurologistes de Langue Francaise* 50 (1952), 503–13. However, I first came across it quoted in *Anatomy of an Epidemic* by Robert Whitaker (Broadway Books, 2010). I have drawn upon Whitaker's excellent book in offering this brief history of chlorpromazine.

7   Elkes, J., and Elkes, C., 'Effect of Chlorpromazine on the Behaviour of
    Chronically Overactive Psychotic Patients', *British Medical Journal*
    2:4887 (1954), 560–5. http://www.jstor.org/stable/20330113

8   Actually there is some dispute as to when Heinz Lehmann first
    started using the term 'antipsychotic'. I've settled on 1961 as described
    in *A Historical Dictionary of Psychiatry* by Edward Shorter (Oxford
    University Press, 2005), 26.

9   I found this chlorpromazine statistic on Wikipedia. Sometimes you
    just have to look stuff up on Wikipedia. (Incidentally, the name
    Wikipedia is a portmanteau. The 'pedia' part of it is taken from the
    word 'encyclopaedia'. The 'wiki' part of it is from the Hawaiian word
    for quick. So: Wikipedia = Quick Encyclopaedia. And I know *that*
    because I looked it up on Wikipedia.)

10 Read, J., Psychiatric Drugs: Key Issues and Service User Perspectives
    (Mind, 2009), 2–3.

11 Russo, J., 'Through the Eyes of the Observed: Re-directing Research
    on Psychiatric Drugs', *Talking Point Papers* 3 (McPin Foundation,
    2018). http://mcpin.org/wp-content/uploads/talking-point-paper-3-
    final.pdf

12 Heres, S., Davis, J., Maino, K., Jetzinger, E., Kissling W., and Leucht,
    S., 'Why Olanzapine Beats Risperidone, Risperidone Beats
    Quetiapine, and Quetiapine Beats Olanzapine: An Exploratory
    Analysis of Head-to-head Comparison Studies of Second-generation
    Antipsychotics', *American Journal of Psychiatry* 163:2 (2006), 185–94.

13 Morrison, P. D., and Murray, R. M., 'The Antipsychotic Landscape:
    Dopamine and Beyond', *Therapeutic Advances in Psychopharmacology*
    8:4 (2018), 127–35. doi: 10.1177/2045125317752915

14 The theory of excess dopamine causing 'aberrant salience' was first
    posited by the psychiatrist Shitij Kapur. For more, read: Kapur, S.,
    'Psychosis as a State of Aberrant Salience: A Framework Linking
    Biology, Phenomenology, and Pharmacology in Schizophrenia',
    American Journal of Psychiatry 160:1 (2003), 13–23. doi: 10.1176/
    appi.ajp.160.1.13

15 Morrison and Murray, 'The Antipsychotic Landscape'.

16 Murray, R. M., and Di Forti, M., 'Increasing Expectations and
    Knowledge Require a More Subtle Use of Prophylactic
    Antipsychotics', *World Psychiatry* 17 (2018), 161–2. doi:10.1002/
    wps.20517

17   For a critical view of biochemical theories in relation to psychiatric drugs, see (or see again, since I've already recommended it): Joanna Moncrieff, *A Straight Talking Introduction to Psychiatric Drugs* (PCCS Books, 2009).

18   For an easy-to-read and informative discussion about antipsychotic medications, consider the pamphlet *Making Sense of Antipsychotics* produced by the mental health charity Mind. https://www.mind.org. uk/media/4703393/antipsychotics-2016-pdf.pdf

19   I've written about some of the damaging effects of hospital bed closures myself. You may wish to read my article: 'Mental Health Care: Where Did It All Go So Wrong?', *Guardian*, 25 January 2014. https//www.theguardian.com/society/2014/jan/25/nathan-filer-mental-health-care-where-did-it-go-wrong

20   For a fascinating paper by Robin Murray and colleagues dissecting the notion of a schizophrenia brain disease, read: Zipursky, R. B., Reilly, T. J., and Murray, R. M., 'The Myth of Schizophrenia as a Progressive Brain Disease', *Schizophrenia Bulletin* 39:6 (2012), 1363–72. For more on the macaque monkey study in particular, see: Dorph-Petersen, K. A., Pierri, J. N., Perel, J. M., Sun, Z., Sampson, A. R., and Lewis, D. A., 'The Influence of Chronic Exposure to Antipsychotic Medications on Brain Size Before and After Tissue Fixation: A Comparison of Haloperidol and Olanzapine in Macaque Monkeys', *Neuropsychopharmacology* 30:9 (2005), 1649–61.

21   Marshall, M., Lewis, S., Lockwood, A., Drake, R., Jones, P., and Croudace, T., 'Association between Duration of Untreated Psychosis and Outcome in Cohorts of First-episode Patients: A Systematic Review', *Archives of General Psychiatry* 62:9 (2005), 975–83. doi:10.1001/archpsyc.62.9.975

22   For NICE guidelines on Early Intervention services, see: https://www.nice.org.uk/guidance/qs80/chapter/Quality-statement-1-Referral-to-early-intervention-in-psychosis-services

The Keyholder, the Non-keyholders and the Voices

1   The quotations from Philip Corlett are taken from my interview with him in December 2018. For more on his research, read: Powers, A. R., Bien, C., and Corlett, P. R., 'Aligning Computational Psychiatry with

the Hearing Voices Movement: Hearing Their Voices', *JAMA Psychiatry* 75:6 (2018), 640–1. doi:10.1001/jamapsychiatry.2018.0509

Leaving the Heartland

1 For an illuminating discussion of the WHO findings, I recommend Chapter 3 of *Crazy Like Us – The Globalization of the American Psyche* by Ethan Watters (Free Press, 2010).